Body Eloquence

The Power of Myth and Story to
Awaken the Body's Energies

by
Nancy Mellon

with
Ashley Ramsden

Foreword by Donna Eden

www.BodyEloquence.com

Energy Psychology Press
Santa Rosa, CA 95403
www.energypsychologypress.com

Cataloging-in-Publication Data

Mellon, Nancy.
    Body eloquence: the power of myth and story to awaken the body's energies / Nancy Mellon with Ashley Ramsden ; fore-word by Donna Eden. — 1st ed.
        p. cm.
    Includes bibliographical references (p.   ) index..
    ISBN 978-1-60415-028-5
    1. Organs (Anatomy)—Popular works. 2. Organs (Anatomy)—Mythology. 3. Energy psychology. I. Ramsden, Ashley.
II. Title.
    QM26.M45 2008
    612'.028—dc22

2008011465
© 2008 Nancy Mellon

Cover design by Karen Kane, www.CuriousSky.com
Typesetting by Karin Kinsey
Typeset in Perpetua and Calligraphic
Printed in USA
First Edition

10 9 8 7 6 5 4 3 2 1

CONTENTS

Foreword

Who has not sat in rapt wonder at the body's inner workings, hearing about how the immune system mobilizes a posse to attack an invader or that a single cell undergoes some 100,000 chemical reactions per second? What intelligence orchestrates these micro-dramas within us?

Body Eloquence is a thrilling read, guiding us into the cornucopia of poetic relationships that reside in the human body. Its thesis is that every organ embodies a purpose and has an influence that goes far beyond its biological function. Every organ is as vitally connected with psyche and spirit as it is with blood and oxygen. As every organ contributes to your life story, it embodies a specific theme, holding its important piece in the cosmos' great mysteries.

The heart is not merely a remarkably durable pump. It is the embodiment of good will, sending nourishment to every fiber of your body and being, the receptor of "heart-to-heart" connections with those you love, and the organ of an openhearted embrace of the world around you. But if its influence is too strong, if you are too openhearted, you are overly vulnerable to the slings and arrows from within and from without that cause heartache, that break the heart and its spirit. If its influence is too weak, if you become small-hearted, you move through the world with the miserly constrictions that reflect a body in which not enough oxygen can flow.

The kidneys are not just organs of purification, filtering the blood and transporting toxins from our bodies. As Nancy Mellon shows, they inhabit the deep interior worlds within us, nourishing our life stories with philosophical depth and transcendental understanding. The pancreas and spleen not only process and balance the blood; people who are strong in this energy bring a sweetness to life and impart stability to others.

For every organ, this book provides not just these broad-stroke simplifications, but a depth and richness that will help you comprehend the organ and its themes in ways that will change how you think about not only your body and its parts, but also your place in the universe. By understanding the great themes of life according to each organ when it is in perfect balance and harmony as well as when it is not, the big questions of psychology and philosophy become palpable, soul-sized dramas set in the tangible theatre of a body trying to thrive.

Nancy Mellon draws together science, medicine, mythology, and healing traditions in telling the story of every organ and the energies (which travel throughout the body along pathways known in traditional Chinese medicine as meridians) that govern it. You will relate to these stories intuitively and instantly, and you will be changed. I will request of all my students and suggest to all the practitioners of the healing arts I know that they read this beautiful and profound exposition.

The eloquence of your body and its organs is the voice of creation speaking to you directly and uniquely. This book shows you how to decipher its language. It also instructs you in how to engage in rich dialogue that informs, directs, and heals your body and its organs. Storytelling goes in both directions. Not only does every organ have a story to tell, your body also resonates with the sounds of the stories conjured by your imagination. Even your cells respond. Whereas our inner talk is usually *from* our mind *to* our mind, story speaks to every level of our humanity. As Nancy Mellon explains, great storytellers reach out "with their voices to respond to the secret dreams and struggles of human beings and all living things."

This is a book that teaches you about the great storyteller that dwells within each of us, addressing at once the grand themes of Heaven and Earth and the perpetual conflicts among our organs, the product of our day-to-day adjustments to the planet. It is a book that teaches you to be attuned to the spectacular dramas within, finding the stories that complete what is unfinished, that right what has been wronged, and that move us further along, and with greater consciousness, on this journey we call life.

Donna Eden
Author, *Energy Medicine*
November 2007

Acknowledgments

This book could not have been written without the inquisitive genius and generosity of Bob Cooley, and those who attended his Meridian Stretching Center in Boston, Massachusetts, from 1991 to 1997. Bob's stamina for exploring each of the territories in this book during that time greatly informed and inspired my own. Ashley Ramsden's countless tales, spun with warmth and amazing ease, demonstrate how stories resonate simultaneously within body and soul, mind and spirit. The hospitality of various learning centers, especially Emerson College in Sussex, UK, and many inspiring students, clients, friends, and colleagues continue to help this work evolve. John Docherty, Antoinette Botsford, Harvey Zarren, Sharon Sassaman, Sidora Ziegler, Jeff Imperato, Sonia Story, Davina Muse, Zoe Weil, Katrina Lewers, Ramsay Raymond, and Equanimiti Joy generously read the book as it evolved. Dirk Kelder and Livia Morvay also offered many helpful insights and technical skills.

When what is presented here does not accord with traditional teachings or with your personal beliefs, I hope that you will nevertheless enjoy and benefit from these explorations, and further them. Many Eastern and Western spiritual and medical teachings, especially those of Rudolf Steiner, inspired me to question how nature and the greater cosmos weave within every detail of the human form, and awaken consciousness. In this study of the body's wisdom, I am also very grateful for my experiences with eurythmy, yoga, storytelling, healing through the arts, and energy medicine — and to my family and dear friends near and far who are not already mentioned here.

Introduction

For thousands of years, the storytellers and philosophers of India have shared the image of a boundless net stretched across the skies above the palace of Indra, the supreme ruler of the gods of ancient India. At every crossing point of this net shines a jewel. Each unique jewel mirrors every other jewel. The tale of Indra's net tells us in mythic pictures what science is discovering today: that all is connected within us and outside us in the greater universe. This book invites you to experience your body as a whole through stories, and to discover that each part is in continuous communion with all the others, with your whole soul, and with far-reaching spiritual dimensions of who we are all together in an evolving universe. It is a celebration of the very evolved and inspirational community within us all.

Because every part of the body is closely connected with every other part, this book is intended to be read as a whole. As humanity grows closer together, everyone's body listens to the unfolding human saga in order to discover new pathways to mutual acceptance and understanding. Our organs are gathering places of wisdom, continuously cooperating below the surface of our consciousness. I believe that it is very important for us to listen more closely to all of them. Organized and perfected over long cycles of time, they are the physical-spiritual crucible for our personal and communal human evolution. Each organic pattern can awaken vast new understanding and inspiration for relating to ourselves and to each other.

Another purpose of this book is to develop understanding of how storytelling is a healing art that can draw out the innate wisdom within us. Stories make us more aware of ourselves as part of feeling, creating, laughing, crying, curious, courageous humanity. Together they have a cumulative effect, broadening our inner knowing, our compassion, and our sense of self. They can also help us to nourish the body's natural intelligence by speaking directly to and from the intricate weave of our bodies.

Human consciousness is a whole-body experience. By working through the chapters of this book, you will learn to commune directly with the vast intelligence at work within you. As you collaborate more consciously with the creative genius by which your bodily life evolves, thrives, and heals, your relationship with yourself and others will evolve with it. No matter with what satisfaction or dismay you see yourself in the mirror, you can perceive all your parts, and everyone else's, with new wonder and respect. The body is far more than something attractive to be adored, or to be exercised in health clubs; more than a chemical genetic factory to be studied; more than an apparatus with parts to be taken out and replaced or repaired in a bustling hospital or clinic. I believe that the mechanistic view of the body is but one step in human awareness.

Each chapter in this book is devoted to an organ and begins with a description of its physiological role in the body, presented from both Eastern and Western perspectives. The chapters present the fundamental meridian energy patterns known for many centuries in traditional Chinese medicine (TCM), followed by simple physical exercises to experience these fundamental energy patterns that stimulate a more artistic, creative, and globally oriented relationship with life. Each chapter also explores the soul physiognomy that resonates with each organ territory. Examples of individuals who embody these organic characteristics, often drawn from my therapy practice, are described, together with stories from many traditions that illustrate themes arising from each organ.

The "Transformational Storytelling" portion of each chapter offers you an affirmation to support the health of the organ and invites you to summon and to activate the storyteller within you that resonates with each organic territory. Transformative story patterns that have served storytellers for centuries portray the dance of positive and negative energies through protagonists and antagonists, and illustrate how bodily awareness can enhance the art of storytelling and support self-development. Each chapter also includes a variety of creative exercises for exploring the energies of each territory, as well as dance, music, and yoga asana selections to further expand your awareness.

The organs described in this book are living entities that carry us ingeniously through our lives. Each of these inner bodily territories communicates with great sensitivity with our unique individuality. Each shapes and forms lively relationships with the others as it mediates specific energies. A hugely responsive flowing, drumming, cascading, leaping conversation is continuously taking place amongst them and influences our daily conversations with ourselves and others. We sometimes sense these organic relationships in our dreams and in imaginative pictures in our waking hours. They lift us up or weigh us down as they give rise to inner characters and landscapes. As soon as we connect intentionally with one or another of these shaping energies through creative expression, we enter zones of excitement and risk.

You will feel more immediate affinity with certain of the organ realms and their stories, and less with others. Yet as you incorporate all the chapters in this book into your everyday perspective and let them stimulate your own creative expression, you can profoundly change the way you experience your body and soul. Like reagents in a chemical experiment, their different characters and plots can rearrange your attention, bodily energy, and spirit for life.

World conditions today, more than ever before, summon us to greater awareness of ourselves as whole and evolving human beings who are able more fully to awaken to the vastly dynamic wisdom that intimately plays within each of us.

Storytelling Is a Healing Art

When I was a teenager, I worked one summer in a hospital to explore whether or not to pursue a career in medicine like my parents and my great grandmother, who was one of the first women MD's in the U.S. As I was helping babies to be born, I was also privileged to attend an amazing operation that allowed a man who had been deaf for many years to hear again. This was a turning point for me. I realized then that I wanted spend my life opening listening, and bringing new life to the spoken and the written word.

My journey with transformational storytelling began in an international Waldorf school that nurtures the arts as the foundation for learning. Standing before a class of children each day to deliver stories from a global curriculum, I quickly found proof that well-spoken stories build life forces. Sometimes as I made up and told stories, and looked out to see the children's eyes shining as they lit up from head to toe, I would feel my whole body resonating like an orchestra. Later, when I became less involved with classroom teaching and was completing my training as a psychotherapist, I was invited to work in a clinical setting with adults who were recovering from a broad range of chronic physical and emotional illnesses. I decided to experiment with storytelling, and I was fascinated to see positive results right away.

This launched me into a surprising new career. It was the beginning of the many storytelling classes, workshops, and courses I have continued to give during the past two decades. I often open these sessions by saying to tired and discouraged people: "We are going to work with that part of your mind that is creative and loves stories. Every one of us has the ability to make up wonderful healing stories. During our time together, you will tap into that part of yourself that is a playful yet very wise storyteller. Spontaneous storytelling resembles dreaming, yet allows you to be awake and to participate in the healing process." During these sessions, as dull eyes brighten, cheeks lose their pallor, and backs straighten, I observe with great wonder and pleasure how illnesses readily respond to the energy of the creative self and its inherent drive to health on the physical, emotional, mental, and spiritual levels.

My goal from the start is to encourage movement in a healing direction. "Slowly take some good, deep breaths," I say. "As you inhale and exhale, sense a listening space in your heart. Let your whole body relax and listen. Breathe with your whole body, as if you are a healthy child. As you relax more deeply, your critical analytic mind can rest and your creative mind will awaken to speak in ways that may surprise you. Great storytellers reach out with their voices to sense the dreams and struggles of human beings and of all living things. Like countless storytellers before you who have experienced the healing and organizing power of stories, you can breathe beyond the barriers of mere reasoning and clock time, into depths of creativity."

As participants relax and listen more openly, I explain that imagination thrives when it is given specific tasks. I invite them to imagine that they are opening a large and magnificently illustrated storybook. "On the first page of your book, envision a hero or heroine who embodies a quality that you esteem in other people and in yourself, such as courage, kindness, contentment, or playfulness. Visualize the picture in detail: how the character is dressed—notice the colors, shapes, and textures. In what era and environment does he or she seem to be living?"

Traditional tales often end with a positive sense of celebration. To encourage group participants to liberate their hopes, I continue: "Protagonists often set out to find greater love, health, power, joy, and happiness. In your beautifully illustrated book allow your imagination to show you a picture of a place of fulfillment and happiness. Let your breath take you to this place. Is it by the sea, a mountainside, a valley? Is it in a town or a city, or perhaps on another planet? As if you are a child studying a superb illustration, notice the plants, creatures, and architectural structures. What fragrances, sounds, and colors do you associate with this picture? Enjoy the details you see or sense, and remember them well."

A sense-filled search for positive beginnings and endings stimulates creativity and allows worries and doubts to rest. Truth contained in the core of the personality emerges, penetrating sinews, muscles, heart, and soul with wisdom beyond ordinary conscious thought. In my workshops, these hopeful endings are usually shared with a partner, whose only task for a while is to listen openly like a child and to share in return. Afterward the groups sit together, savoring the images that have emerged. Stimulated by storytelling imagination, genuine empathy and understanding flow more freely. A sense of endings and new beginnings flourishes. A woman who had been depressed for as long as she could remember imagined with wonder a family that expressed much love for a sadly neglected child. The woman had found within herself at last a positive imaginative response to her childhood yearning for love. An exhausted man gratefully resonated with the landscape his imagination presented to him: a quiet green cove where his hero would live in peace and harmony. A depressed father, after describing a king who was very devoted to his subjects, clearly saw himself making more time to spend with his daughter.

Harnessing the imagination to the body can reveal unknown obstacles, and awaken new solutions and resolutions to health. When they are pictured in the context of a story, physical symptoms often lessen, or even disappear completely, sometimes permanently. Having stimulated positive, creative beginnings and endings, I then encourage other rhythmic story patterns. When working with the body, I give yet another task to the storymaker: "Even your most troubling problems or illnesses can be seen through the eyes of your imagination as a landscape or a character. Include your physical or other struggle in your story either directly as a character or as a sound, color, or landscape."

Using this technique, a woman emerging from a prolonged depression envisioned herself as a beautiful fictional character: "Penelope was curled up in an earthen den. She had been there, it seemed, for a long time. She would awake, and sensing that nothing had changed, she would return to sleep. She was wrapped in her long, shining hair." A man who was resolved to release himself from a habit that had clouded his life since childhood pictured a story character in a dark cave, bound hand and foot with ropes. As his character began to move and call for help, the ropes turned into dust.

BASIC STORY ELEMENTS

Myths and stories often resonate with specific internal processes. This reliable pattern invokes well-being and resilience in every cell of your body:

Setting Out: The protagonist sets out in quest of greater love, strength, justice, wisdom, and happiness.

Trouble: One or more obstacles and/or antagonists interfere with the journey.

Help: Wise and benevolent help comes, often giving a gift.

Positive Ending: The protagonist fulfils the quest with joy and celebration.

THE POWER OF CREATING AND SHARING A WHOLE STORY

I have never met anyone who was not able to tell a whole story from beginning to end. You might think you can't, but in working with the storytelling exercises in this book, just go forward and tell your story in honor of the multitudes of courageous storytellers who have gone before you. You will be following a reliable pattern utilized by countless storytellers throughout the world.

Stories can provide paradigms for the process of healing. The main character in many fairytales and myths sets out on a journey and eventually finds new love, health, power, strength, and happiness. When the time comes for your protagonist to be in deep trouble, especially remember to keep breathing. During the story you will tell, allow the richness and truth of your soul-life to bring forth help whenever it is needed.

In stories, anything is possible. Animals speak. Stones and gems with benevolent powers work magic. Angels may appear in many forms and disguises. A tree or flower may say exactly what a character needs to hear in order to proceed on his or her journey. Welcome whatever helpers are presented to you by your imagination, even if they greatly surprise you. Allow these kind, ingenious, powerful helpers to work with you. At the end of your story, remember the positive ending that you have just made up. Let your ending be a celebration.

TRANSFORMING BODY AND SOUL THROUGH STORIES

In one of my storytelling classes, an especially profound response to the storytelling process came from a woman who had recently been diagnosed with cancer. At the start of the session, I suggested she might bring her illness as an imaginative picture into the story. Though distraught and pale, stretched out on a couch beside her worried storytelling partner, she nevertheless willingly followed the directions. First she envisioned her protagonist, and then a positive ending. Still collapsed and weak after she shared her first images, she listened closely as the others also shared theirs. When it was time to assemble a whole story, she sat upright beside her partner and launched into the telling. When her protagonist reached the obstacle zones, she brought her cancer directly into the story. She described it vividly as an amorphous dragon-like creature with shifting eyes and edges.

Then an angel came into her story. It fought with the monster, and prevailed. The woman triumphantly rose to her feet and told her story to the group, recounting the battle that occurred in her story. Her voice became increasingly clear. Her face shone brightly as she spoke and she seemed to have shed many years. Bewildered and filled with joy, she asked, "What happened? I was telling a story and then I was filled with light. I have never experienced anything like this before." A concurrence of events had brought from deep within her a comprehensive spiritual, mental, emotional, and physical transformation. She experienced a profound improvement in her health by accepting the help that came through the gates of her imagination.

How do stories bring about such transformation? Was this a once-in-a-lifetime experience? As if to help me explore these questions, a young woman who had been diagnosed with leukemia attended the class in the early days of my experiments with storytelling as a healing art. She, too, worked with extemporaneous storytelling in a larger group and afterward asked to continue the process. During her private session, she confided that she sensed there was an emotional story behind her physical illness. I knew very little about her personal history at that time, but I wanted her to have as positive and healing an experience as possible during our brief time together. I asked if she would like to create a new story and place in it the greatest obstacle to her health.

In a meditative reverie, she told in metaphor the story of recurrent physical abuse that had occurred several years before the onset of her illness. I offered to write down her story as she spoke. When I finished reading back to her, she exclaimed through her tears, "This is not a bad story!" Speaking at the imaginative level helped her to remember her real-life story and to speak openly through pictures about the traumatic experiences she had endured. Following the rhythmic story pattern had helped the images arise freely. In a brief time, she was able to revisit her own pain, and to realize through the story she told how unawakened were the people who had caused it. This was a strong response that she had not expected.

"I have just now really experienced a healing from hearing how my story ended," she said quietly. "The abuses happened out of ignorance. When one gets to a certain level of consciousness, there is no way one could do anything like that."

Flooded with forgiveness for the ones who had caused her so much distress, she said that she wanted to let go of her illness completely and to begin a new life. She sensed with more clarity than ever before that her illness had been connected with her feelings of helplessness, fear, and rage. She clearly knew that she needed to be of service to others as a part of her healing path. Expressive and aware, she felt more focused and free, and new energy flooded through her whole being. A few months later, I learned that there was no trace of leukemia left in her body and that she had begun pursuing a new career in the healing arts.

How I Began to Learn the Organs' Stories

Such comprehensive healing experiences inspired me to continue exploring the power of storytelling. I had worked for many years with the ancient Greek system of diagnosis and healing through the elements of earth, air, water, and fire. I wanted to expand my knowledge to include the traditional Chinese medical system, with its cosmic understanding of the human body that is thousands of years old. On this quest, in 1991, I met Bob Cooley, a brilliant and hilarious former mathematics instructor who was busy at that time developing his Meridian Flexibility System in Boston, Massachusetts. Slowly and tenaciously, Bob had put himself back together after suffering a life-threatening accident. As he vigorously explored the ancient sciences of yoga, traditional Chinese medicine, kinesiology, and modern psychology, I discovered how specific muscles and meridians (the body's energy channels identified in Chinese medicine) connect with specific organs to support the whole human being. After a few early morning sessions at his Meridian Stretching Center, I wanted to understand the healing dynamics I was witnessing in Bob and in the people who gathered at his studio.

As Bob guided us into astonishing experiential group research, he shared his questions and discoveries, encouraged individualized exercises, and helped us to push further. Stretching this muscle group and that, and attending to the effect, my whole life became more flexible and aware in each organ domain. I began to realize that our fresh inquiries into the energy patterns of the body were adding present-day picture language to the ancient imaginations that are taught through traditional Chinese medicine. As a great variety of often completely unexpected thoughts, images, and sensations tumbled through us, I frequently could not scribble notes fast enough to record all that was happening.

Practicing various yogic stretches, I discovered that intensive stretching along specific meridian lines sometimes released whole personality patterns from within me. In Bob's studio and my home practice, as marvelous and fascinating casts of distinct realities emerged spontaneously from within me, I acted them out to experience and understand them more fully. As my consciousness expanded with schizoid glee, I studied these patterns quite methodically from within myself. My ability to experience these distinct personalities was enhanced because, as a writer and teacher of creative writing, I often meet surprising characters that develop during the creative process. As a performing artist, teacher, and puppeteer, I had directed, written, and acted in many plays. As a psychotherapist specializing in the healing power of the creative arts, I was also interested in all possible therapeutic benefits.

Yoga is a path of integration. After a particularly vigorous session of stretching one early morning, I stood up to catch my breath. A rush of new awareness flashed through me as I recognized that all the world's story patterns and characters are inscribed within the human body, and that someday I would write this book.

In 1992, I attended a storytelling performance of British-born Ashley Ramsden during one of his tours in the United States. He was busy embodying a broad realm of characters through the spoken word, and becoming well known as the extraordinary storyteller he is, with a growing repertoire from around the world. By that time, I had worked with storytelling as a healing art for many years and Ashley invited me to teach at the storytelling school that he had recently founded at Emerson College in Sussex. Eventually, his curiosity, too, was piqued by the resonance between stories and the body.

In January 2000, as the twentieth century ended, we began working together in search of the stories that resonate with each organ realm. This book is the result of our quest. As I gradually described to Ashley what I was experiencing through the various organs, he told stories that resonated with them from his immense memory trove. Exploring the reciprocal patterns of organs and stories often felt like learning to recognize unfamiliar planets or constellations. As the search continued, many workshops and courses about the body's eloquent design evolved. We marveled with others at how all the organic realms generate and respond to particular stories, and how nature and the greater universe support the storytelling process when it is in the service of truth and well-being.

Each organ carries out its own function diligently and enjoys its life. Each is a gateway of spiritual activity with its own intelligent mind-soul that is very sensitive to whatever is going on in our lives. In this tour of these inner organic realms, as there is such a need for greater heart wisdom in our present world, let us begin with the heart.

1

Cheerful Mediator: The Heart

The Persian poet Hafiz wrote: "Your heart and my heart / Are very, very old friends." Even as we go about our sometimes jangled and dissonant lives, we resonate with one another. Whenever our hearts meet warmly, their circulating power permeates our whole selves with a reassuring sense of well-being. When we meet someone who lives fully in the heart's majestic realm, we naturally feel awe and gratitude. At the other extreme, those whose hearts seem cold or empty tend to be puzzling or frightening.

Place your right hand slightly to the left of your breastbone to sense the four chambers of your heart enjoying life together. Blood that is low in oxygen pours into the right atrium, the right ventricle, and then into the lungs to recharge with oxygen. Returning to the left atrium, oxygen-rich blood gathers momentum in the lower left ventricle to spread out into the thousands of miles of arteries, veins, and capillaries in your body. Tilted slightly forward, this especially hardy and active left ventricle inspires the phrase "I mean this from the bottom of my heart." Heartfelt positive thoughts and feelings churning through the chambers of our hearts awaken us to its primordial sunny magnitude and origins. Like every organ, the heart is embraced by celestial influences and carries profound memories of its evolutionary journey. During embryonic development, the earliest form of the human heart floats above the forming head, like a miniaturized version of the Sun above the Earth. Only gradually does the embryonic heart descend inside the fetus, to beat with its intimate and dependable warm inner radiance.

In traditional Chinese medicine (TCM), meridians, or energy lines, run throughout the entire human body. These energy lines are not unlike energetic currents, often referred to as

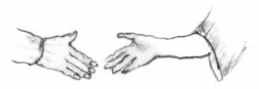

A Warm Handshake

"ley lines," that crisscross the globe. Expanding the usual Western image of the work of the heart within the body, the TCM perception of the heart includes cosmic energy moving through the body that is not wholly dependent on the physical heart and blood circulation. Chinese physicians perceive the heart meridian as an energy channel that radiates through the heart downward under the arms and across the inner elbows into the palms of our hands and the inside tip of our little fingers.

A warm handshake and a story do wonders to strengthen the heart. As we meet others with a vigorous handshake or clasp our own hands together, warmth streams through our arms. We may feel the heart's energy filling us with good will. As we shall see throughout this book, such seemingly simple gestures as a handshake release specific energy patterns. Through increasingly relaxed and alert body awareness, the energy patterns of each organ territory of body and soul presented in this book will become familiar to you. As they do, you will recognize them in yourself and in others with increasing empathy, like sunlight illuminates an outer landscape.

Heart-strong folk are sanctuaries of comforting acceptance. They imbue others with the warmth that circulates so strongly within them. As they resonate with the task at hand, their serenity helps to bring about negotiations and flowing reconciliations. One evening I found myself unexpectedly in the presence of an enlightened guru and was astonished to find my heart growing gently synchronous with his. After a time, it seemed that my heart contained every human being who has ever been, with ample room to spare.

The inner circulation of heart-strong people gives them embracing, well-rounded perspectives. In stressful or dangerous situations, these folk tend to remain levelheaded, and to speak with calm honesty. As they resonate with the heart's mission to bring sturdy, harmonious flow to life within them and for others and their natural surroundings, they gravitate

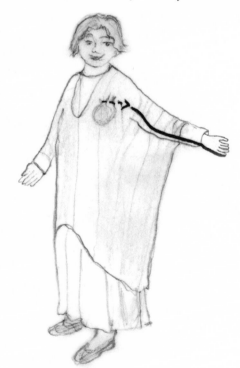

The Heart Meridian

toward body-based work, meditation, and relaxation techniques. They tend to generate heartfelt utopian visions.

THE STRIVING HEART

Kirk, an elderly friend, manifests a well-developed heart personality and physiognomy. When Kirk retired from his college career at age seventy, he felt called to become a storyteller. In his athletic youth, with his strong chest and muscular arms and his love for physical strength, he gave himself to his beloved American ideals and signed up to be a U.S. Marine. Yet active service in Korea soon caused him to feel revulsion for himself and his fellow soldiers.

When Kirk returned to the United States after his soul-wrenching combat duty was over, he resolved to transmute his anger and become a warrior for peace for the remainder of his life. He became a college professor, at the same time working as a counselor, volunteering in hospices to help the dying and their families, in battered women's shelters, and with families suffering from AIDS.

I was in the audience when Kirk told his first story in public. Soon after he had emerged from major heart surgery, he resolved to explore storytelling and learn to express all the caring warmth he felt in his heart. His charisma and his tale opened the hearts of everyone in the auditorium. When he finished, we all sat back, deeply moved. Encouraged by our response, he soon began to speak about "throwaway" people and others he wanted to rescue by weaving them into stories. Whenever he told his tales, an atmosphere of compassion and love pervaded the room. He soon found other venues for his stories, and his confidence grew.

Several months later, Kirk was among the people who came to my home to explore storytelling as a healing art. He gradually learned to trust the whole group. On the day of the final group presentations, Kirk waited, listening to the others. He had decided to tell the story that as a soldier had most devastated his heart, and wanted to wait until it was pitch-dark outside. The former marine began to speak in the candlelit room, and in the course of his story, he screamed forth a horrifying rape scene he had witnessed. After fifty years, the experience that had been suppressed so long within him pierced through the darkness to the stars.

This was a turning point for Kirk. He had liberated his heart's story of bitter disappointment and rage at his comrades and himself. Afterward he found that for the first time he was able to feel new and profound compassion for himself and for other veterans. Kirk now contributes to group therapy sessions in veteran hospitals. When he tells his tales, he sits sturdily on a stool. Through his presence and gestures, his pauses and repetitions, powerful yet gentle heart forces stream forth to all who listen. On Kirk's answering machine, his outgoing message offers an expansive sense of time: "Leave your message. There's no rush. You can turn time into a flower." He wants to help everyone prevent heart problems.

The Wise Heart

Countless stories convey the reconciling, stabilizing wisdom of the heart, and encourage the heart's steady warmth and vigor. All our organs confer and work together, constantly in touch with one another, yet separate and individual. They play cooperatively like musical instruments in an endless concert. A tale from Borneo portrays the heart in conversation with some of our other vital organs.

❦

Who is More Important?

A very long time ago, when all the parts of the body were just beginning to get together, they gathered for a conference. They were trying to decide which was most important.

The eyes were the first to speak. They said, "It is clear that we see into everything. We recognize what is coming. We are the ones who perceive the truth."

Said the ears, "We are more important."

"You? What about me?" said the mouth. "Everything comes through my door."

"Fools," said the feet. "We carry you everywhere."

"What about me?" said the nose.

"Let's face it," said the sexual organs. "If it weren't for us, you wouldn't be sitting here at all."

On and on went the debate. The different parts of the body argued amongst themselves for long days and nights. Finally, all the parts were exhausted. Then they heard a voice that seemed to come from very far and also very near, inside all the other voices. They recognized it as their own, and yet not their own. It whispered and also thundered within them.

"My brother and sisters, have you forgotten my pleasure in your existence?" This was the voice of the heart speaking. "How can we exist without any one of us?"

All the other voices knew that what the heart had spoken was true, and they were filled with joy and peace.

❦

Following the Heart

A healthy heart generates comforting physical strength. It paces itself, and does not rush. It shapes our physiognomy and sense of direction, and also influences our speech. A hard-working woman decided to walk for three weeks during the summer along an old pilgrimage route on the coast of Spain. Over many stressful years, she had acquired polyps on her vocal cords, and speaking was very painful. Now she sensed her need to revisit her past in order to release anger pent up within her, which she had absorbed from her troubled family. Carrying only a light duffle, she went alone.

"My body wanted to feel the truth. My brain wanted to know the whole story," she explained.

She walked steadily. Her heart filled with fresh energy. After a week, a ferocious temper fit discharged from deep within. Soon afterward, a refreshing melody sang through her. She was amazed to hear herself singing simple words of love. As her heart opened, more and more fragments of the family saga that had been suppressed were reconciled within her. By the third week, her throat felt better. She had found a fresh speaking voice and, as she walked along, many songs flowed freely through her.

EARTH'S HEARTBEAT

Through the ages, conditions that stress both individual and communal hearts continuously call for healing story and song. How can we encourage the harmonizing strength of the heart to speak more fully and more often?

⟶✦⟶

Fences or Bridges

Two friends who had been neighbors for years had an argument and stopped talking to one another. Soon afterward, one of them found a kind-looking young man on his doorstep, carrying a box of tools.

"Do you have any jobs I can help you with?" he asked.

The man decided to trust him. "See that wide ditch? My neighbor plowed it deep between his property and mine, and flooded it from his upper pond. I want you to go out there and build me a tall fence so I won't have to look at his property any more."

Then the man set out to get some supplies in town. When he returned at sunset, his eyes opened wide and his mouth fell open. There, instead of a fence, stood a bridge spanning the ditch. It even had handrails.

His neighbor crossed the bridge with both hands outstretched and said, "What a fellow you are to mend our friendship with a bridge."

As the carpenter put his tools in the box and hoisted them onto his shoulder, both neighbors begged:

"Why don't you stay?"

"I'd like to," he replied, "but there are so many more bridges to build."

Over the years, the friends took time to cross over and visit one another, and to keep their bridge in good repair.

⟶✦⟶

Not long ago, human beings expressed the rhythms of their hearts more organically than we do today. They experienced the sun as a warm drumbeat within them. In present-day culture, it is increasingly challenging to find the way into these healthy rhythms, yet many storytellers and musicians succeed. I was recently introduced to a drum made out of wood cut from an old tree. This tree had been chosen because its trunk had grown indented into a heart shape. The Native Americans who stretched white deerskin over this huge mother heart drum meet regularly with friends to drum, chant, and share their stories.

Among the tales cherished by the Cherokee nation, one tells about love turned to anger and then restored through powers beyond ordinary means.

❦❦❦❦❦

Strawberries

Long ago, in the early world, there lived the first man and the first woman. They lived together as husband and wife, and they loved one another dearly. But one day they quarreled. Although neither could remember the reason later, the pain grew stronger with every word that was spoken, until finally, in anger and in grief, the woman left their home and began walking away to the east, toward the rising sun.

The man sat alone in his house. The anger left him and all that remained was terrible grief and despair.

A spirit heard the man crying and took pity on him. The spirit said, "Man, I have seen your woman walking to the east toward the rising sun."

The man went after his wife, but he could not overtake her. Everyone knows that an angry woman walks fast.

"I will go ahead and see if I can slow her steps," said the spirit, who soon found the woman walking, her footsteps fast and angry and her gaze fixed straight ahead.

There was pain in her heart. The spirit saw some huckleberry bushes growing along the trail, and made the bushes burst into bloom and ripen into fruit. But the woman's gaze remained fixed. Her footsteps didn't slow. She looked neither right nor left, and she didn't see the berries.

The spirit caused the trees of the forest to burst into bloom one by one and ripen into fruit. But the woman's eyes remained fixed, and still she saw nothing but her anger and pain. Then the spirit caused a green carpet to grow along the trail starred with tiny white flowers, and each flower ripened gradually into a berry that was the color and shape of the human heart. As the woman walked, she crushed the tiny berries beneath her feet. Their delicious aroma rose to her nostrils. She stopped and looked down, and she saw the berries. She picked one and ate it, and she discovered its taste was as sweet as love itself.

So she began walking slowly, picking berries as she went, and as she leaned down to pick them, after a time she saw her husband coming behind her. The anger had gone from her heart. All that remained was the love she had always known. So she stopped for him, and together they picked and ate the fruit. Finally, they returned to their home, with a new taste of peace and happiness.

⸙⸙⸙⸙⸙

Some of the finest European tales collected by the Brothers Grimm portray the transformational power of the heart. Enlightened storytellers sought to strengthen the hearts of their listeners through rhythmic plotlines. Though the hero of "The Queen Bee" is teased and called a "simpleton," nothing stops him from heeding the sunny generosity of his own heart.

⸙⸙⸙⸙⸙

The Queen Bee

In the early part of the story, Simpleton is dozing and making music peacefully by the home stove, yet he misses his older brothers who have left home. He senses they are struggling in the great world without him. At last he finds them and the three brothers begin traveling along together.

Soon their footsteps bring them to an anthill. The two elder brothers want to see the little ants scurrying in terror, carrying their eggs away. But the youngest brother says: "Leave the creatures in peace. I will not allow you to disturb them." Then the brothers go onward and reach a lake where a great number of ducks are swimming. The two older brothers want to catch a couple of ducks and roast them for dinner, but Simpleton says: "Leave the creatures in peace. I will not suffer you to kill them." At length they come to a bees' nest in which there is so much honey that it is running down the tree trunk. The elder brothers want to make a fire beneath the tree to suffocate the bees in order to take the honey, but their simple brother again stops them, saying, "Leave the creatures in peace. I will not allow you to burn them."

The three travelers arrive at a castle where stone horses are standing in stone stables and where nothing is moving with life. They go through all the empty halls of the castle until they come to a door with three locks. In the middle of this door is a little window-pane, through which they see a gray-haired old man sitting at a table. They call him once, twice, but he does not hear. When they call him for the third time, he gets up and opens the locks. He wordlessly conducts them to a handsomely spread table, and after they have eaten and drunk, he beckons them to sleep. Next morning the little old man shows the eldest brother a stone table, on which three tasks are inscribed: Find all the princess's pearls, find the golden key to her chamber, and choose from three sleeping princesses the one who can best rule the realm. Completion of these tasks, according to the stone inscription, will deliver the castle from its enchantment.

Neither of the older brothers is able to succeed with even the first task and both become lifeless stone statues, joining countless other gray statues in the chilly stone halls of the castle. Finally, it is Simpleton's turn to try the tasks. He seats himself on a stone and weeps, thinking that what his brothers could not accomplish, he will not be unable to accomplish either. But soon, to his wonderment, the king of the ants whose life he saved from his brothers' cruelty comes with five thousand ants and, before long, the little creatures have got all the pearls together in a heap. The second task, finding the key to the bedchamber of the king's daughters, also seems impossible to Simpleton because the key is at the bottom of a lake and he does not know how to swim. Yet when Simpleton comes to the lake, the ducks he saved from his brothers' greed dive down and bring the lost golden key to him. The most difficult task remains: identifying which of the three sleeping daughters of the king shall be the true queen. The queen of the bees whose nest Simpleton saved from fire helps him discover his true bride.

And so the whole castle is delivered from its enchantment, and those who had been turned to stone return to life. Simpleton marries the princess whose heart is most pure, and after her father's death, they rule together. His two brothers marry her two sisters.

◦━◦━◦

Like many a heart-centered story that churns our feelings in the direction of love, "The Queen Bee" skillfully dramatizes the blood's circulation through the four chambers of the heart. The whole story moves steadily in a recurring rhythm of three trials resolving like the fourth beat in a musical phrase. The anthill is the first testing place for the three brothers, the duck pond the second trial, the honey hive the third. Simpleton's strong will and loving kindness bring the brothers safely through these trials.

Without intending to, we can lose touch with our heart's trusty rhythmic flow. Disappointed and hurt by our fellow human beings, we may retreat into stony slumber or fume with anger. Yet as the gray embattled castle of the mind lets go, pure childlike innocence can freely radiate its sunny warmth.

Transformational Storytelling
Heart Affirmation
My heart is filled with a ceaseless song of love.

Basic Heart Story Dynamic
Anger becomes unconditional love.

Heart Protagonists and Antagonists

Heart protagonists (characters who support heart health) are unconditionally loving, majestic, unprejudiced, and cheerful. They are given to timely, warm, and wholehearted action to support others.

Heart antagonists (characters who express heart dysfunction) are whiney. They avoid conflict and are excessively concerned with comfort. They can be angry, passive, slothful, and oblivious of others.

Basic Story Elements

Myths and stories often resonate with specific internal processes. This reliable pattern invokes well-being and resilience in every cell of your body:

Setting Out: The protagonist sets out in quest of greater love, strength, justice, wisdom, and happiness.

Trouble: One or more obstacles and/or antagonists interfere with the journey.

Help: Wise and benevolent help comes, often giving a gift.

Positive Ending: The protagonist fulfils the quest with joy and celebration.

SUMMONING YOUR STORYTELLER

Heart-strong storytellers plant themselves before their audience like sturdy oaks. Their presence is a transfusion of kindness that strengthens the inner circulations of their listeners. These storytellers are robust and warm, like an oven full of baking bread. They tend to clothe themselves with wholesome simplicity and to receive their audiences gratefully, hoping for listeners as openhearted as they are. Their tales strengthen compassion and hope; their speech and their gestures are measured and rhythmic. They may gesture before they speak, opening the way for compassion and confidence to pulse and circulate, just as blood vessels open the way for blood to pulse and circulate throughout the body. The voices of heart-strong storytellers are reassuring, conveying a mood of comforting ease. As they open the heart, they invite the smart and busy mind to rest.

Exercises to Explore and Balance the Heart

Focus on the organ and its meridian lines. Practice openness. Shifts of awareness can happen on the physical, mental, and spiritual levels as you explore stories connected with each organic territory and awaken your own storytelling abilities.

Let your heart speak. Allow yourself a peaceful space of time. Sit down with a piece of paper and write out these lines: "I am your heart. For years I have been wanting to speak with you." Listen well to your heart and write down what you hear it saying.

Reflect on areas of your life in which your heart feels at home. Invite your heart into one of those areas from which it feels excluded. As the poet Rumi wrote: "Everything has to do with loving or not loving."

Heart story dynamics. If someone is deprived of love, the heart sends messages to the whole body. Imagine a character who lives in its strong, gentle rhythmic beat and sway and is peacefully journeying through a sunny landscape. Even a brief imagination of healthy heart energies can liberate energy that may have been blocked for years, and release healing pulses. Hearts contract and withdraw when they sense love is lacking. Protective shadows gathered around the heart can be expressed as an antagonistic dozy character who avoids conflict. Tired and discouraged hearts lack suppleness. They bump lethargically without a sense of direction. In loveless circumstances, the heart can collapse painfully or slowly break. All of these heart conditions can be portrayed through your story characters.

In a two- or three-minute story, let a heart-strong protagonist and a dysfunctional antagonist meet. Surprise your mind. For example, you might imagine a hearty traveler whose way is blocked by a conclave of dull giants or chilly robots. Antagonists in stories and in life stimulate positive action. As your story continues, let help come to support your protagonist. Although your mind may resist this positive plotline, let love, warmth, and joy triumph at the end of your story.

Every day, news stories challenge and devastate our hearts. Yet as we summon the storyteller who lives within us, we can create and live stories in which heartbreak turns in a more positive direction. Although events shatter love, hearts mysteriously mend. To feel the authority of human resilience within you, try this for yourself: At the end of a difficult day, light a candle. Seek a feeling of heartfelt warmth for a few moments; then tell a story to yourself, your family, or a friend or two. The language of heart stories is usually straightforward, sturdy, and compassionate, as in the examples you have read in this chapter. Enjoy the rhythmic warmth and regularity of which your voice is capable. As your words synchronize with your heart, unexpected feeling might arise and radiate. Tap your foot slowly to regulate the pace of your speaking, or use your hands or beat a tambourine or drum.

Shape characters to strengthen the heart. Perhaps you know someone who, like Kirk, the troubled soldier in this chapter, is quietly consumed with rage at world conditions. Create for this person a story that transforms rage into powerful compassion.

Portray the light of your heart in a story. A well-known Middle Eastern tale tells of a traveler who comes in a dark forest to a cottage full of candles. A very old man welcomes him, saying, "Here live the souls of all people."

"Then may I see my own soul?" asks the traveler amidst all the glowing light.

The old man shows him a lamp that burns with only a wisp of flame. The traveler tries to snatch another's oil, but the old man gently restrains him. "The lamp will glow brighter when you strengthen your heart."

Then the cottage disappears and the traveler resumes his journey with new resolve. Continue this story.

Personal and community development. Imagine a person whose heart has been taken hostage and hidden away, like the Tin Man's in L. Frank Baum's *Dorothy and the Wizard in Oz.* Describe the chill in its absence. Create an adventure story to rescue this heart and restore it to its rightful place.

Synchronize and strengthen the heart in a group. To explore and strengthen the heart's four chambers that continuously function together, work in a group of four. Commune with your own internal music and its universal rhythms. As you place your fingertips on neck or wrist to feel the pulse beat of your blood, a sense of harmony will build in the group. As the heart gathers strength, listening opens. Gradually synchronize your pulses, swaying and perhaps drumming on thighs and chests. Slowly rise up as a group to dance. Then sit down again, taking turns to create a story in which a heart is sorely challenged, yet prevails against all opposition and thrives. First let your inner storyteller present you with a protagonist who embodies the heart's strengths. Take this character triumphantly through three obstacles, like Simpleton does in "The Queen Bee." As each member of the group contributes to this adventure, the others hum, clap, softly tap, or drum to keep rhythm as the story unfolds.

Speak from the heart. You may already be experiencing how stories open a sense of connection between yourself and others and bring light to negativity, as when sunlight dispels darkness. Parents often ask me how to bring out painful family stories for their children. I tell them that no matter how many problems their family group carries, speak from the heart. Children listen for our feelings and attitudes at least as much as to our words. They are watchful to see how we connect with our feelings as we tell them about ourselves and others.

The heart's holiness. In many ways, this book is a manual for love. To express the heart's realm, I often go to a large heart-shaped pond near my home. Imagine, create or locate a space to which you can go to honor the heart's wisdom.

Expanding Heart Awareness Through Dance, Music, and Yoga

Dance

Turning ceremoniously to north, east, south, and west, pound your feet as if to a steady drumbeat. Then stand firmly grounded and reach out with your arms and hands to embrace the whole world. Open your palms wide and radiate energy outward from your heart center through all your fingers as you press your heels down. Place your hands together at your heart and breathe in and out slowly. Relaxed full-body breathing allows the heart's warmth to rise into consciousness as it opens more fully. Now slowly lift your hands straight upward to the twelve o'clock position and then allow them to descend to your sides as if your arms and hands are warm, radiating beams of sunlight. Turn these basic gestures into an ongoing dance built on a rhythmic base of four beats. Include all the directions in your dance.

Music
Pachelbel, Canon in D Major
Handel, Air from *Water Music*
Bach, Arioso from Cantata no. 156
Mendelssohn, Wedding March from *A Midsummer Night's Dream*
Leonard Bernstein, "One Hand, One Heart" from *West Side Story*

Yoga asanas (Sanskrit names in italics)
Full-Body Breathing *(Pranayama)*
Downward Facing Dog *(Adho Mukha Svanasana)*
Sun Salutation *(Suryanamaskar)*

2

Artist in Residence: The Small Intestine

The gracefully looping tube called the small intestine is a collecting place for gutsy transformations. This softly flowing connection between the stomach and large intestine measures about twenty-five feet in a mature adult body. Peering into its lively iridescent lining with a microscope, we would see its intricate cellular layers with millions of leaf-like structures called villi, each one with millions of microvilli surrounded by lymphatic ducts and nodes. As the small intestine tastes and tests nutritional substances, it gradually pushes them onward toward the large intestine. Meanwhile, like an alchemical laboratory, it takes on other ingredients for processing. As it transmutes nutrients, it can also fire up as much as two-thirds of our immune activity.

As with every other part of the human body, the continuing health of the small intestine depends on many subtle connections with the creative world within and around us. Storymakers, storytellers, and all creative people are continually communing with the vast, vibrating transformative activity that surrounds the Earth in waves of wind, water, and fiery light. Over an immeasurable period of time, this elemental tumult has coiled itself with microcosmic ingenuity and efficiency into the human form.

Western medical science acknowledges that the shimmering snakelike form in the hold of our bellies contains more than meets even the microscope-aided eye. The ancient Chinese, observing how the body maintains its order, identified the small intestine as an extensive energy pattern. Its meridian begins on the inside of the tip of the little finger and moves across the hand and wrist upward and behind the shoulder to the center of the back. Here it divides to join with heart, diaphragm, and stomach energy before entering the small intestine. Other branches rise along the sides of the face to the outer corners of the eyes and to enter each ear.

To feel the refining, spontaneous, fiery strength of the small intestine, place both your hands on your belly and breathe deeply. Lift and expand your heart as you feel its pulsing dance. Then press your littlest fingers together, while pressing your forearms together and lifting them too. Continue attending to your breathing until your eyes and ears relax. Have you ever found your little finger lifting as you hold a spoon or sip your tea? Whenever the little finger turns upward and outward, this indicates that the artful and exciting peristaltic heat of the small intestine is well turned on within you.

SEEKING THE DIVINE THROUGH ART

Through exercise you can experience how the small intestine contributes to the upward flow of cerebrospinal fluid, giving us refined, gutsy intelligence, and the drive for passionate creative expression. Its heated activities inspire love of the arts as they enliven our visual sensitivity and ignite transformative and intimate expression in music, theater, film, and design. Its quickening energies bring forth a uniquely expressive alchemy of body and soul, whether in poetic wordsmithing, music, sculpture, or flower arranging. An active sense of beauty often results in deep-seated repugnance toward the sluggish, unaesthetic aspects of industry, commerce, and bureaucracy. Even today, some visual artists spend much of their time making paints and gathering various ingredients

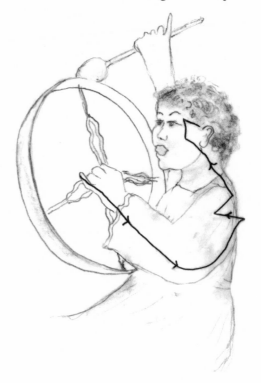

The Small Intestine Meridian

to seek different hues and shades. As in the past, they grind and mix stones or the roots and blossoms of plants, turning raw materials into luminous hues for their palettes and canvases. They invent wonderful brushes, and take pleasure in selecting just the right substance to make something beautiful. They seek expression to which the whole life-body can cry "Yes!"

Some of my favorite people are quirky impulsive artists who love the wonder of the creative process. Artistically expressive by necessity, for their health they have to heed Mother Teresa's counsel to "make something beautiful for God." For them, anything can be composed into an artistic event. With the impulse to make art out of truth, their creative expression can sometimes appear facile, superficial, and frenzied, until it finds a deep sense of courage. Lalla, a fourteenth-century mystical poet of Kashmir, fully realizing the liberating fire in the realm of the small intestine, wrote:

> *I didn't trust it for a moment*
> *but I drank it anyway—*
> *the wine of my own poetry.*
> *It gave me the strength to tear down the darkness*
> *and cut it into little pieces.*

Struggling to transform the destructive impulses they experience within them, these natural artists design rooms and clothes and arrange beautiful prints and graphics to express the many layers they sense in their personalities. They produce films of striking intensity.

A friend of mine whose personality expresses the energy of the small intestine realm lived many painful years of depression and low self-esteem, her creativity suppressed while she let others sabotage her brilliantly clear inner spirit. As she discovered how to fire ahead and leave the past behind, she gradually claimed more time and space for her creativity to flower. Now she fills her house and garden with her own fabulous creations to commemorate her true feelings. She builds shrines to the Great Mother. For her, everything has richly varied viewpoints and is capable of processing, reforming, and even completely transforming. In her hands, satin, foil, and lace turn into dazzling creations. She spends hours foraging for raw materials at the local recycling center, reclaiming rusty throwaways to turn into beauty. She welds and wires sculpture out of copper and scrap metal, or she hand-sews politically sensitive words into books with soft fabric pages and whimsical bindings, embroidered inside and out with fiery fibers. Her work expresses the energy of digestion and transformation, the urgency of her intestinal fortitude.

FINDING BEAUTY EVERYWHERE

Small intestine personalities love visual beauty. They collect, organize, and bring forth images to share, hoping their own pictures or their galleries will uplift and transform. My elderly friend Ethelwyn burnished colored stones with an electric tumbler. Firing them with colored glass, she formed over the years thousands of brilliant birds and butterflies. New as the morning sun, she arose each day with the glee of a child to open her kiln and behold these creations. Twice a year, she would sell or give them all away, to make room for more.

Another friend is an intensely loving and creative teacher. In her home and at school, she is surrounded by projects, paint tubes thrown into a basket, books, calligraphy, pets, children, and countless collections of fascinating items. Strong daughter of Sarasvati, the Hindu goddess of the creative arts, she emanates beauty and creative mettle. She thrives on the stress of having so many people depending on her creativity.

When the volatile emotional heat of the small intestine flares, a reasonable person often loses perspective. Although most people have bouts of artistry, some who are strongly centered in the small intestine live daily with artistic bouts. Many such people experience particularly intense and recurring cycles of creation and destruction. A man painted every day for years, hanging canvases in every room of his house or leaning them against the walls. He regularly called his friends to take them away so that he had room to paint more. One day, he began to feel so deeply repulsed by his creations that he built a huge bonfire and burned all his remaining work. As the ashes were smoking, he left his house to search for a new and higher path of creativity. Eventually, after seven years, he circled back and began to paint in a completely new way.

A depressed woman on a healing journey wanted to remember how creative she had been in her younger years. Summoning courage in front of a group, she said: "Once when I was a child, I closed all the doors and I turned the music up until the room felt completely tumultuous. Then I danced with the beauty and power of the music, and everyone I imagined as my audience became the music with me!" As she spoke her memory, she stood more upright. Color came into her cheeks; her eyes sparkled. Remembering and activating our creativity stimulates the small intestine and can free us from even the most negative dramas of our lives. Our creativity transforms us. Time opens up as destructive impulses become grist and fodder for making something beautiful. Hysteria, addiction, and depression can turn into creative genius that completely surprises our darker impulses.

Backed-Up Creativity

It can be extremely frightening if benevolent creative energy collapses or backfires. In my therapy practice, my clients and I relive their biographical struggles in order to push on with their lives. One day a sensitive artist who was feeling abandoned and unloved came pounding with both fists on my office door, in a full-blown fit of hysteria. Moaning and shouting, the woman fell into the room at my feet. "Help me! Help me!" she cried. "I can't go on with my life. I'm going to kill myself."

At that moment, I was very grateful to be familiar with the hysterical negativity that arises from small intestinal stress. I put my hand compassionately on her back, and asked her the question she had forgotten to ask herself, "What happened to your creativity?" This had the desired effect of reversing her energies.

Within a few moments, her face was flushing brightly. She sat bolt upright as she described one of her many long abandoned artistic projects. She took a huge breath and began to tell me what she needed to do. A few days later she returned, smiling and excited. She had enlisted hearty support from her friends and already had brought to completion two of the creative projects that had backed up within her.

Repressing the Muse

What happens when creative fire is dampened, and does not spark through the darkness of our inner lives? When the creative studio is taken away, the playroom boarded up, paint boxes and musical instruments hidden away in dark drawers and corners, we suffer the stifled creativity in ourselves and others.

Even a brief story can neatly and powerfully contain the extreme emotions embodied in the small intestine: repulsion and attraction, desolation and hope, anxiety and joy. During a five-minute writing exercise in one of my "Storytelling as a Healing Art" workshops, a woman astonished herself as she discovered the creative strength hidden within her. Her story of blocked creativity began:

> Once there lived a queen with her many children. She waged life, not war, and all her realm was alive with creative fire. Delightful creations poured forth from her hands and those of all her subjects. When she sang, dancers danced. When they danced, she matched her music to their rhythms. Damask curtains and lace hung in layers at the windows and deep carpets cushioned her footsteps. Light played upon her walls in rich colors, along with the laughter of the children and serving maids, and so life went on though the upward spiraling years. Boats burst into her harbors, bearing songs and spices from diverse directions of the sea. Her life was replete with jugglers and trapeze artists flying through trees. One day, however, an enchantress invaded the realm, quietly at first, depressing the queen's servants with her steely gaze. At last she gained control of the queen herself....

But by the time the woman had finished her story, the queen had magnificently regained her authority.

Multitudes of stories express in picture-language the creative ingenuity of the small intestine. Intestinal alchemy is portrayed with brilliant luster in a tale about a powerful old Chinese artist.

⁂

Wang-fo

Old Wang-fo was making slow progress on the roads of the Kingdom of Han because he stopped so often to observe the natural world. He loved to portray nature in his paintings. For him nothing seemed worth buying except brushes, pots of lacquer, ink, and rolls of silk and rice paper. His disciple, Ling, carried a sack full of his master's sketches, bowed over as if he were carrying the heavens. For Ling the sack was full of snow-covered mountains, torrents in spring, and the face of the summer noon.

One fateful day, Wang-fo was summoned to the Imperial Palace where the emperor sat on a high throne in his meditation garden. Surrounded by Wang-fo's paintings, this emperor had been brought up in solitude, never feeling free to express himself. When he was sixteen years old, at last he was allowed to look at life outside the palace for the first time, but found it far less beautiful than the master's paintings. With tragic bitterness, the thwarted young emperor cried: "This world is nothing but a mass of muddled colors, thrown into the void by an insane painter, and smudged with our tears."

The emperor's desire for beauty beyond this world turned to disgust at the harshness of reality. He conceived a punishment for the painter, whose artistry had filled him with such awe. He decreed the artist's eyes that saw such beauty be burned out and that the hands that expressed it be cut off. But first he slaughtered Ling, the artist's faithful servant. Then, upon a sign from the emperor's little finger, two eunuchs respectfully brought forward the unfinished scroll on which Wang-fo had outlined the image of the sea and the sky. Wang-fo selected one of the brushes that a slave held ready for him and began spreading wide strokes of blue on to the unfinished sea. A fragile rowboat grew under the strokes of the painter's brush and now occupied the entire foreground of the silken scroll. The rhythmic sound of the oars arose in the distance, quick and eager like the beating of wings.

Then by the magic of the old master's artistry, Ling arose and helped his master into the spirit boat. As the sound of rowing filled the room, strong and steady like the beating of a heart, Wang-fo finished the painting and the emperor, leaning forward, a hand above his eyes, watched Wang's boat sail away in a golden mist and disappear. The painter and his disciple vanished forever on the blue sea that Wang-fo had just created.

✦❧✦❧✦

IGNITING CREATIVITY

As necessity turns us into audacious artists, it also nourishes and builds us up. The small intestine part of the psyche is rooted in the riddles of creation and destruction. To live primarily from these roots for a whole lifetime can be extremely challenging. Like the great Hebrew kings David and Solomon, many artists swing between poles of intense creativity and of self-destruction. An infested gut can cause the mind to seethe with a surreal ferment of dark images. When this happens, the immune system reacts with aches, pains, depression, and chronic fatigue. A woman who had been tormented by her dreams for many years quite suddenly connected with the positive energy of her small intestine. A surprising flow of images revealed feelings she had never before dared speak. As she put these images together into a story, an unexpected healing process was ignited.

The Snake in the Fire

Once upon a time in a cave, a small fire grew into a huge snake, but then it sank down again and disappeared. Suddenly, it shot out of the cave again and blew fire over the sky. The people from the nearby village fell back in great anxiety. But a village boy fearlessly entered the cave.

"Foolish snake, why are you so moody?" he demanded.

A powerful voice responded, "Snake Queen has thousands of years of life within her. She fulfills a heavenly task."

Then the snake showed herself in all her glory, filling the sky with her magnificent fire. On the top of her head, a small glowing cross of white gold shone in all directions. The village boy heard her say in a commanding voice, "You have no permission, by the law of this cross, to demean me!"

He bowed, thanked the Snake Queen, and left the cave repeating over and over to himself, "I will show respect for all."

After this passionate and fearless flow of creativity, the woman who created the story had unexpectedly found her "guts." An upright magnificent spirit had arisen from within her. She felt more powerful and well than she could remember. In the days that followed, her story became a guide that helped her to claim her power, and to change her life.

As creativity strengthens the immune system, it sometimes leads to sublime personal transformations. When searching for stories that express the dynamics of the small intestine, I rediscovered Sir Richard Burton's *The Arabian Nights: Tales from a Thousand and One Nights.* His nineteenth-century translation fills sixteen volumes. These Indian, Persian, and Arabic stories were collected along the Asian Silk Route during the tenth and eleventh centuries.

In the fabulous frame story at the opening of the Arabian Nights collection, a sultan falls into the deepest despair to which a human being can descend, and through the art of storytelling, Scheherazade saves his life, her own, and many other lives as well. Many other great story collections exemplify the healing power of storytelling, among them Chaucer's *Canterbury Tales,* Lady Murasaki's *Tale of Genji,* and the Indian classic *Panchatantra.* In fourteenth-century Italy, Boccaccio compiled the *Decameron* stories told by a group of young men and women who withdrew to a country house, where they whiled away many weeks telling one another stories to protect themselves from a plague that killed thousands of people.

Healing the Vengeful Sultan

In ancient Arabia there lived two royal brothers. The elder, Sultan Ryhar, ruled in the south and the younger the kingdom in the north. One day Sultan Ryhar invited his brother to visit him. The younger brother prepared for his journey by gathering silks, slaves, and concubines to offer as gifts to his brother. Then he set out on his journey in the cool of evening. But when he was outside the gates of his city, he remembered a jeweled box he wanted to give to his brother. So he returned to the palace. As he approached his royal bedroom, he heard the sound of laughter. Creeping closer, he saw his wife carousing on his bed with a greasy cook.

He was furious. "If this goes on when I am within sight of the palace, what might this woman do while I am away?" He drew his scimitar, stormed into the bedroom, and with one blow cut the two of them into four pieces.

Then he returned to his men and went on with his journey. As he traveled, he became sick and pale. When he arrived at his destination, his elder brother had prepared a feast and celebration for him, but the younger brother was not interested in food. His brother sent for physicians. After several weeks, the elder invited his brother to go hunting with him, but he refused. Instead he wandered distraught through the palace. As he strayed from room to room, he happened to look through a small lattice window onto one of the courtyards below. There he saw his older brother's wife carousing with slaves.

He later revealed to his brother what he had seen. Learning of his wife's unfaithfulness, such madness overcame Sultan Ryhar that he too slayed his wife and vowed to repeat this revenge forever. Each day a new maiden was sought and found to satisfy his destructive desire. He spent the night with her, then had her executed the next day. So it went, night after night, until mothers and fathers fled with their daughters and prayed that his rule would come to an end.

Now the sultan's chief vizier had two daughters. Scheherazade, the elder of the two, loved to go to the marketplace to listen to storytellers. She was witty, wise, well read, and well spoken. She retained all the stories she heard. She also studied sciences and all the other arts. For a long time, she had heard of the king in his madness marrying in the night and killing in the morning. She suffered deeply from what she heard.

One day she went to her father and said, "Father, will you grant me a wish?"

The vizier loved his daughter and said, "Of course, my dear. Anything."

"Then let me marry the sultan."

The thunderstruck father replied, "You know what will happen?"

"Father, if you do not give me permission, I will go to the king myself."

The vizier knew his daughter well enough. Once her mind was made up, there was no changing it. So he went to the king and told him what his daughter desired.

"You know that I have made an exception for you and your daughters," said the sultan.

"My Lord, this is what my eldest desires."

"Very well, I will marry her, and tomorrow she shall die."

But Scheherazade had a plan. She said to her sister, Dunyazade, "Tonight after the king has taken what he wishes, I will send for you. Turn to me and say, 'Please, my sister, tell me one of the wonderful stories you have often told me at night before we went to sleep.' Perhaps this will save us."

So that night the king married Scheherazade. Just as they were about to fall asleep, she turned to him, "Please, sire, let me say farewell to my sister, before the dawn comes, and with it my execution."

The restless king said, "Send for her."

Soon Dunyazade knelt at the foot of the bed and said, "Please, my sister, tell me one of the stories you have so often related to me before we slept."

Scheherazade asked permission of the king, and then she started. Time passed. Dawn approached. She told of a fisherman, a king turned to stone, and a magical genii. Just as light broke over the horizon, she stopped.

"Well, what happens next?" demanded the king.

She replied, "My lord, with apologies, I can only tell stories at night."

The king agreed to wait until the next night. When night came, she finished the story and began another. The king also wanted to hear that one through. Again, as dawn broke on the horizon, she hadn't quite finished it. He had to wait again for the next installment. So it went on, night after night. Each morning, the vizier would turn up with a winding sheet for the dead body of his daughter, but she always greeted him, radiantly alive.

Scheherazade told the sultan stories portraying men and women's tricks and deceptions, and the twists and turns of fortune. She skillfully wove all manner of stories of common folk, sailors, pirates, princes, and thieves; stories of the wise, the cruel, the ambitious, the foolhardy; stories of animals who speak and scheme; stories of travel, adventure, loyalty, love, friendship, heroism, betrayal, envy, and every human foible and grace imaginable.

As the sultan listened to her succession of tales, he was nourished every night by her voice, and by the power of her glowing sensitivity. His tormented soul began to repair. Through the three long years that Scheherazade told the thousand and one stories, the storyteller and the desperately wounded king sometimes also talked and made love. The heat and fire of their relationship gradually warmed and opened the king's heart.

On the one hundred and forty-fifth night of stories, the once miserable king looked at his clever companion tenderly and said, "Your words are delicious in their newness. They combine to lead me in a milder way."

After one thousand and one nights of stories had passed, Dunyazade asked the sultan, "Do you still wish to kill my sister?"

"How could I possibly?" he replied. "She has touched my heart. She has revealed to me the true meaning of love and wisdom." And the sultan went to Scheherazade and asked, "Will you forgive me for all I have done?"

"My liege, there is nothing to forgive, for you are no longer the man you were."

Then Dunyazade entered his chamber with three children, one walking, one crawling, and one sucking.

"Who are these?" the king asked.

"These, my lord, are your children."

The sultan, fully released from his torment, joyfully sent for his brother, who fell in love with Dunyazade. Together they celebrated a double wedding, and a scribe was engaged to write down the stories so they could be passed on to everyone. It is said that whoever hears them will be blessed forever.

⋙⋘⋙⋘

As the sultan immersed himself in Scheherazade's wisdom, in time his balance was restored. His connection with the archetypal world quickened. He did not so much understand the stories as absorb them into his soul, like mother's milk. Scheherazade is the archetypal healing storyteller. She applied the art of storytelling with shamanistic elegance, to meet head on the sultan's suffering and miserable destructive impulses. For a thousand and one nights, her own life, and the lives of many others, depended on her transformative skill. The wit and self-esteem she had developed by listening to stories in the marketplace allowed her to digest and transform the king's confusion and hysteria. As the king was swept along and held by Scheherazade's tales, the steadiness of her heart, combined with her wit and fire, helped him to discover a more complete humanity within him.

SCHEHERAZADES TODAY

A mother who joined one of my storytelling as a healing art circles resolved to make a new version of an old legend. I told the group an old story in which the young women of a village were sacrificed one by one to a terrible dragon. With this, all the mother's protective instincts flared. She was surprised as her words and gestures took on unaccustomed intensity as she told us her own version of the old legend. In her version of the old story, one of the villager's courageous daughters went to the mouth of the dragon's cave and shouted fearlessly, "*I am here!*" Then the girl began to sing beautifully to the fuming dragon in his dark lair, and to tell the dragon a story. Like Scheherazade, she left the story unfinished, promising the dragon that she would return the next day. And so the brave girl returned home safely from that first visit to the dragon, and many times thereafter. The mothers in the group loved this cliffhanger. Together they communed with the girl's power, glowing with determination to bring the story to a very satisfying ending. "And to this very day," their story ended, "the daughters of the daughters of the daughter still go to sing heartily and to tell stories to the dark and burning chaos in the cave. And so they protect themselves, and the dragon too."

TRANSFORMATIONAL STORYTELLING

Small Intestine Affirmation

Beauty, truth, and love flame through me.

Basic Small Intestine Story Dynamic

Self-denigration transforms into passion for truth, beauty, and goodness.

Small Intestine Protagonists and Antagonists

Small intestine protagonists (characters who support small intestine health) are artistic, inspiring, have faith in the universe, perceive with passionate clarity, and draw forth beauty and creativity from themselves and others.

Small intestine antagonists (characters who express small intestine dysfunction) feel abandoned, fretful, depressed, self-contemptuous, and impulsive. They are hysterical in bouts. In a depressed state, they feel inadequate, inferior, and un-nurtured, even desperately suicidal.

Basic Story Elements

Myths and stories often resonate with specific internal processes. This reliable pattern invokes well-being and resilience in every cell of your body:

Setting Out: The protagonist sets out in quest of greater love, strength, justice, wisdom, and happiness.

Trouble: One or more obstacles and/or antagonists interfere with the journey.

Help: Wise and benevolent help comes, often giving a gift.

Positive Ending: The protagonist fulfils the quest with joy and celebration.

SUMMONING YOUR STORYTELLER

Storytellers who inhabit the energies of the small intestine express a fiery creative spirit. They dress with uniquely stylish elegance. Their gestures are graceful and intense. Their words at times may be highly charged with emotion, yet they speak with sparkling poise in flowing streams. They long to express beauty that will transform the hidden depressive darkness in themselves and others and inspire creative endeavors. They are relieved of countless anxieties by allowing themselves to articulate the beauty of a story. Their backs straighten, their hearts spring up and forward, and their eyes sparkle. Sensitive to nuances of color and form, they especially enjoy sharing graphic visual impressions.

Exercises to Explore and Balance the Small Intestine

Imagine your art studio. Imagine a space in which you can freely express yourself, even yelling or howling. Is it by the sea, in a city, on a mountainside, or secluded deep in a forest? What artistic materials would you like to have on hand to inspire you? Now invite your voice to access more of its natural poise and fiery force. Be like a child and investigate your voice and the words of your story or poems.

Speak with passion. Expressive and flexible strength arises from the small intestine as grace under pressure. This flowing inner strength can surprise us by bringing forth a passionate assertion of understanding, a rush of truth. Well-worded impassioned poems and stories fire up peristaltic activity. Think of Scheherazade's swiftly brilliant flow of words. Listen to Rimsky-Korsakov's *Scheherazade* and dance to the surging rhythm of lively peristalsis that is expressed in this music. Dedicate the dance to the well-being of others. Perhaps, like Scheherazade, your creative peristaltic energy may save a life.

Then read a poem or a story that is packed with colorful language and feeling. As you read, experiment with different vocal qualities, making your voice change. Let it droop or drift or hurry. Let it sound dry as flour, or icy cold. Well-spoken words have a muscular upright quality organized around a firm backbone of enunciation and grammar. Spoken with intention, words set up a resonant flowing energy field around us. Although much of the resonance of words may be lost in ordinary conversations, each well-formed word, phrase, and sentence strengthens us, body and soul. Honest, clear speaking enlivens the bones and immune system, helps with circulation, and improves digestion of food and experiences. Retell the story of Scheherazade, focusing on the section in which she confronts her father, insisting that through her creativity she can save the realm. Ask a partner to play the role of her father to provide you with oppositional resistance. Then change roles with your partner.

In an imaginative mode, tell or write a story about someone who, like Scheherazade, is able to speak truth with passion and imagination.

Transformation now. Criticism and misunderstanding often inhibit and constrict our creativity. Sometimes, in a very natural way, our creativity flowers, then droops, dies, and disappears, even for long stretches of time. Imagine that a sculptor is shaping you into an embodiment of someone whose creativity has waned or become blocked. What does this look like? Then let the sculptor portray someone who is experiencing the inspired excitement of creative expression. How does this feel? Now flow slowly from the blocked position into the most creative. Go back and forth a few times, rest, and let this dance transform into a story drama. Let your most creative energies have the final word in your story.

Imagine an ominous destructive force lurking in a cave. Whether a personal or mythic beast or plague, let this be met and gradually transformed. In stories, we can invoke honesty, courage, compassion, and every strengthening virtue. The many years of healing stories I have witnessed attest to the power of keeping an unwavering flame of love in the plot.

Resounding creative mettle. In one of the tales collected by the Brothers Grimm, "Many Furs," a young woman caught in an incestuous battle with her parents escapes from their castle, with the spirited ingenuity that is characteristic of the small intestine. Read aloud this tale, which is sometimes entitled "Allerleirauh," or read aloud another tale that expresses audacious mettle and resilience in very trying circumstances.

Seize the moment. Finding a ready-made story to tell can be like shopping for a garment. Fabulous stories with different styles, fibers, and colors wait to be tried on. An effective approach to finding a story that suits your creative mettle is to dive completely into the creative process, letting a new story come forth spontaneously, accepting the artistic intuitive process. As the subconscious works, the story unfolds. The vibrant soul is connected with a healthy, flowing small intestine. Both body and soul are artists participating in the beauty and mystery of each moment. Place three objects randomly on a table or the floor. Quickly make up a story that connects them. Or with a partner make up a story that you have never told before. Your partner has the task of throwing in random words as grist for your creative process. Allow the fiery creativity of your storytelling genius to accept what comes your way and put it to use. Then swap roles with your partner.

Balance small intestine and heart energies. According to Chinese meridian theory, in order to maintain creative flow, the small intestine balances and heals itself through the warmth and earthy strength of the heart. Imagine that a couple representing the dynamic energies of the heart and small intestine speak. What vows would they declare to one another at their wedding so that they can be themselves and also support their partner?

Expanding Small Intestine Awareness Through Dance, Music, and Yoga

Dance

Let your whole body dance with a feeling of undulating grace. Dance your hands together and apart in a stream of figure-eight infinity signs, your arms and hands dancing freely up and down your torso and above your head. Free your baby fingers, as if they are conducting a great orchestra. Move in figure eights across the floor, turning freely in all directions.

Music
Rimsky-Korsakov, *Scheherazade*
Beethoven, Sonata Pathétique, op. 13
Massenet, Meditation from *Thaïs*
Mussorgsky, *Pictures at an Exhibition*

Yoga asanas (Sanskrit names in italics)
Standing Tree *(Tadasana)*
Head to Knee *(Janushirasana Dandayamana-janushirasana)*
Half-Tortoise *(Arda-Kurmasana)*

3

Willing Servant: The Liver

Wordmakers in many languages have recognized the intimate emotional power hidden in this organ that is so central to our well-being. In Persian, *liver* means "darling." Its old English name was *lifer*. The largest, warmest, and wettest of all organs, the liver busily generates life throughout the whole household of your body and soul. Imagine this as a soft cistern within your torso, shaped against your stomach and colon, your kidneys and adrenal glands. Every iota of your blood supply must journey through it.

The liver filters and neutralizes harmful insecticides, food additives, alcohol, and pharmaceuticals. It vies in splendidly bloody battles with parasites, bacteria, and viruses. Sedatives, tranquilizers, and animal fats surrender to its metabolic genius. It takes on newly invented toxins never before known to the human body. Everything that comes into the body from outside is eventually filtered and washed by the liver before surging forth to further adventures in the wider circulation of the body. On a perpetual health mission, liver-strong blood distributes nutrients and energy exactly as needed to the rest of the body.

The liver's energy feels less earthy than the heart's, less fiery than the small intestine's. Although a healthy liver is able to reconstitute itself in a matter of hours, faster than any other organ, if the lively, buoyant ecology of the liver is disrespected, the whole body eventually suffers. To stimulate its juicy vitality, raise your right arm gently beside your ear and slowly bend to the left. Your right side will feel larger and more open. With your left hand and using a circular motion, gently massage your liver area, tucked under your rib cage. Pat it warmly with gratitude

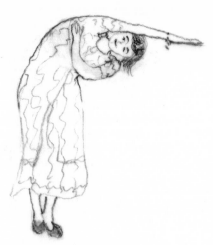

Liver Exercise

for doing its complex tasks. Then lift your left arm, stretch, and massage with your right hand. After only a moment or two of stretching along the liver lines, people typically exclaim, "Ahh, I feel lighter, warmer, more eager for life!"

Through centuries of shared observation, traditional Chinese medicine physicians have seen the liver as a well-tempered strategist bringing will and balance to the whole body. They locate the origin of its flowing energy in the big toe. Try jogging barefoot in a fertile field to feel life teeming in your toes, so often banished into numbing shoes. In fact, the liver meridian flows from the big toe of both feet up over the insteps to the inner knees and thighs and through the genitalia, before connecting with the liver. From there it springs upward

through the lungs and over the top of the head to splash its subtle energies down into the area of the eyes. As it completes its circuit around the mouth, it rouses mirth and bubbling laughter.

Ever ready to sustain a flow of quick energy, the liver absorbs both nourishment and good feelings to make oxygenated, iron-rich blood. As the liver regulates oxygen throughout the body, it creates its own jovial brand of digestive vitality in both body and soul. It sets fresh, oxygenated blood coursing, as if on magical boats, through the thousands of miles of rivers and streams—the large and subtle circulatory channels in the body's mysterious geography. By the time we are born, it is well organized to send blood up through the portal vein from the lower organs of the body. Without a healthy liver, even babies would experience heaviness and swelling in abdomen and legs. Red blood cells stream into the liver from the spleen, manufacturing hemoglobin and an iron will to live. Simultaneously, the liver aids digestion by filtering away stressful substances, such as alcohol and drugs. As we shall see in the next chapter, one of its tasks is to send extra bile to the gallbladder to digest heavy fats.

Awakening to the liver helps me understand from within myself my moisture-rich friends and colleagues who gush

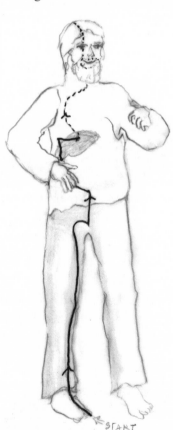

The Liver Meridian

with laughter and storm with tears. As fresh blood arises in the healthy liver, it nurtures outgoing, warmly expressive people of all ages who harbor floods of enthusiasm. As they work in the service of liberty, their effervescent personalities lift us beyond gravity and toxicity like an airline pilot who, with a big smile and controls in hand, carries hundreds of people upward and onward. The multitude that express the liver's health in their personalities have generous, altruistic energy. In keeping with their robust and healthy livers, they eagerly take on challenges. They respond with natural vitality to the liver's call: "Get up and go!" They rouse us with "We're off to see the wizard" or "Let's get together and save the world!" Expressive, gorgeous, and giddy, these folk blow off excessive excitement with peals of laughter. Anything can charge them up emotionally, yet their persistent emotions and laughter can sometimes feel oppressive and controlling.

Navigating life with passionate jovial spirits and infectious laughter, the mirthful sense of mission of liver-strong people can carry them far and wide. As bus and cab drivers, they take lively pleasure in helping us to our destinations and home again. As social workers, they move into impoverished neighborhoods to make sure there is soap and running water, that children have clean clothes to wear, and that mothers and fathers clean up their language and behavior. Like Mr. and Mrs. Santa Claus with rosy lips and cheeks, they may be house-parents for teenagers with special needs, or salespeople who are very good providers. When they are travel agents, their clients may even be inclined to invite them to come along on their trips.

As they actively look out for the welfare of others, such liver-strong folk willingly offer help. They may be accomplished shoppers, like my sister-in-law, who finds just the right gifts for family and friends with uncanny skill. Who do you know that brings the liver's sociable, warm, and adventuresome mission to life? Firemen often inhabit this realm, as do policemen who snare "dragons" in dark places for the sake of a healthier society. They may support Alcoholics Anonymous, where people learn together to face the effects of addiction, drawn to the transformational twelve-step program in which the twelfth step calls for providing service to others. They may insist with strong determination and boundless enthusiasm on cleansing a toxic river or dump site, or on planting gardens and installing sparkling fountains, giving everyone a sense of flowing and refreshing vitality. On collection days, cars and trucks stream into the recycling center in my town with their loads of refuse for sorting and transformation. The center's liver-strong director delights me. He has gradually turned our famously efficient "transfer station" into a convivial meeting place, posted with clear signs and planted with cheerful flowers.

CLEANING OUT THE CONGESTED LIVER

When the natural flow of the liver is held back, gritty feelings can grate against the better self. A few decades ago, it was not uncommon to use the word "liverish" when someone was feeling unwell. A congenial folk remedy says, "Dear, drink a tablespoon of Epsom salts and olive oil with eight glasses of warm water. Take a hot bath, and see what happens in the morning." When I took this advice recently, I expelled precipitously quite a load of gallstones and cholesterol (floating visibly in the toilet bowl). Afterward, though pale, I felt amazingly serene! Epsom salts and oil draw out cholesterol and gravel caught in the liver, moving them on and out. Recovering from the lively peristaltic expulsion of such debris can take a while. A friend who did not know the power of too much Epsom salts caused her family to be sick for a night and a day, ousting the dragon in all directions from every orifice. It is well to experiment with care and respect in your enthusiasm to clean up the liver.

Overburdened livers irritate both soul and body. Unable to act or concentrate, we may leave sentences unfinished and long pauses between words and projects. Our sense of vitality may contract like a tortoise into the hexagonal honeycombs of our liver cells. As the spirit of helpfulness leaves, congestion and inflammation in the liver may brew surly anger, sudden bouts of shouting, and even hepatitis and jaundice. Feuds stored there, like old dragons, may battle below the threshold of our conscious minds, glowering in the form of biliary stones in the cavelike liver ducts. Are you feeling grouchy, or perhaps a little pale and lily-livered? Unwilling or unable to follow through, many eager souls become kvetchy, sour as an unripe plum, like the famed Lancelot when he was unable to perform noble deeds.

We may eventually feel too listless to do anything for ourselves or anyone else. Then a natural hunger develops for chicory, dandelion, or other bitter greens to strengthen anemic will and zest for life. If the liver complains and is ignored, over time it can produce personal and communal insurrections, even delirium, releasing from the liver weirdly terrifying phantasmagoria. I stopped drinking caffeine when I discovered how it overworked my liver. Anyone with an overburdened liver is fortunate to find out, before it is too late, the importance of giving the liver a rest and an opportunity to rejuvenate.

Marit Jarstad, a Norwegian storyteller, healed completely from a serious liver disease by talking with her liver. As a teacher of storytelling, she has told hundreds of people her story:

I became ill with hepatitis B when I was twenty years old. I was in hospital for three months and it took nearly a year before I felt a little better. It became a chronic disease. My immune system was weakened. I tired easily, and through the years, picked up countless colds and bouts of influenza. When I was forty-five years old, a nephew who had just started on his medical studies told me about a doctor whose saga appeared in a prestigious medical journal. When a cancerous tumor the size of a fist was discovered in his head, he was told that he had only three months to live. In this dire situation, he decided to try an experiment. Every day this man meditated on the tumor and imagined it getting smaller and smaller. When three months were up, the tumor had disappeared.

I asked my nephew why I had so many symptoms of hepatitis, since every seventh year all the cells in the body have been renewed. He thought that was an interesting question and told me that the cells with hepatitis gave the image of the disease to the new cells as they died. In this way, my chronic disease continued. He suggested I "talk" to my liver. So I did. Every morning for three months, I told my liver cells, "All is well. There is no danger any more." I must admit I felt a little strange talking to my liver, but after several weeks, suddenly one day I felt well. And I have been well for more than twenty-five years. I took a blood test then those many years ago, and there was no sign of my hepatitis B. The doctor then insisted that I never could have had hepatitis B. Well, well!

Transforming Dragons and Rats

As the liver buoys us, it prompts our most jovial thoughts and service projects. In its good-humored realm, a marvelous uplifting mood predominates. The hero of the old Russian tale "The Fool of the World and the Flying Ship" sets out to seek adventure with only a flask of water and a crust of bread.

He soon meets an old man who asks him for something to eat and something to drink.

"All that I have is yours as much as mine." With those words, the fool's scant nourishment turns into bread and wine.

The wizardly old man says, "Not far down the road you will find a flying ship. Climb on board, and be sure to welcome any fellow adventurers who ask for a ride."

The fool thanks the old man, finds the amazing ship, and soon has risen up and is sailing easily over land and water. Spying a man walking far below him, he swoops down closer for a conversation.

"Take me with you," chuckles the fellow, "and I will bring you merriment wherever you go."

"Then climb aboard," says the captain. And the two rise up and travel on.

The uplifting energy of flying carpets, horses with wings, or helpful flying dragons supply uplift as they embody the liver's mood of merry transport, in league with the gallbladder, moving to subdue, cleanse, and transform anything pernicious that enters the body. To the best of its ability, the liver ingeniously applies itself to a particular toxicity. It strives continuously to turn irritation into enjoyment, and three hundred intricately woven facial muscles into smiles. Neutralizing threats with aplomb, it can bubble forth in luminous hoots of joy and laughter. Within the disciplined bounds of the English nanny tradition, Mary Poppins, who often travels with a magical umbrella over the rooftops of London, also brings about wildly sensible fun. This nanny does not waste time with low self-esteem. Living the high alchemical mission of the liver, she ingeniously dispenses with whatever dims a healthy zest for adventure.

Heroic characters that express the liver's energies can put off physical satisfactions and comforts, like Miguel de Cervantes' chivalric Don Quixote de la Mancha in seventeenth-century

Spain. The great Don longed to relieve distress "in every corner of the universe." Full of rich feeling, this sublimely humorous knight dreamed constantly of grievances to redress, wrongs and injuries to remove, and abuses to correct. An inspirational caricature of the liver's noble mission, he fought inner battles with invisible and visible powers as he sallied forth into toxic arenas to give his whole self, irrespective of his own troubles and skill, to remedy the injured world. Among our many present-day heroes, Michael Moore, in his films *Bowling for Columbine* and *Fahrenheit 9/11,* takes on some of the most serious issues of our time with a marvelous mixture of joviality and unstoppable determination, while moving countless others to similarly life-enhancing deeds.

Robert Browning's story-poem *The Pied Piper of Hamelin* also vividly expresses the liver's immune activity. The sprightly piper introduces himself to the dignitaries of the town of Hamelin, which has been overtaken by a plague of rats:

> *Poor piper as I am,*
> *In Tartary I freed the Cham.*
> *Last June, from his huge swarm of gnats;*
> *I eased in Asia the Nizam*
> *Of a monstrous brood of vampyre-bats:*
> ....
> *If I can rid your town of rats*
> *Will you give me a thousand guilders?"*
> *"One? Fifty thousand!" was the exclamation*
> *Of the astonished Mayor and Corporation.*
> *Into the street the Piper stept...*
> ....
> *And ere three shrill notes the pipe uttered,*
> *You heard as if an army muttered;*
> *And the muttering grew to a grumbling;*
> *And the grumbling grew to a mighty rumbling;*
> *And out of the houses the rats came tumbling.*
> *Great rats, small rats, lean rats, brawny rats,*
> *Brown rats, black rats, gray rats, tawny rats,*
> *Grave old plodders, gay young friskers,*
> *Fathers, mothers, uncles, cousins,*
> *Cocking tails and pricking whiskers,*
> *Families by tens and dozens,*
> *Brothers, sisters, husbands, wives—*

Followed the piper for their lives.
From street to street he piped advancing,
And step for step they followed dancing,
Until they came to the River Weser
Wherein all plunged and perished!

The colorful and captivating musician rid the town of vermin, as he had promised. Yet the greedy mayor and his corporation preferred to use their town coffers to indulge themselves. So the piper laid his jovial pipe to his lips and went to work once more. This time, instead of rats, all the children, except one lame child, followed the piper out of the corrupt township. They founded a fresh tribe, who presumably do a better job of keeping their word and helping one another.

A lame woman who had suffered much abuse in her childhood was deeply touched by the cleansing mission of the Pied Piper, and the children's mood of unstoppable pleasure as they moved beyond the stagnant town. She went ahead to create a new ending for the poem in rhymed verse that portrayed the lame child in the poem catching up with the other children, and being warmly accepted by them.

Seizing Life with Enthusiasm

The liver supports the will to participate in life. In an adventuresome mood, not unlike the Piper's, a middle-school teacher decided to set out on an imaginative journey with her class of twelve-year-olds to teach them world geography. For an entire school year, she related every subject to fanciful travels that took them from their school to the Amazon River, through the jungles of Brazil all the way to the high peaks of Nepal, and full circle back again to their hometown. Their flying carpets included imaginary trains, buses, camels, winged elephants, and donkeys. No barrier interfered for long with their forward momentum. If some students were held back in imaginative delays, other student travelers, eager for more excitement, freed them. Everyone kept a diary, and all year long, enthusiasm ran high. "Let's go!" was their shout. The students and their teacher helped people in distress in imaginary adventures at each stopping place. They became adept at spelling and writing in different languages as they familiarized themselves with different cultures and coinages. At the end of the school year, parents, grandparents, and even a local travel agent attended their coming-home ceremony, as they shared with the whole school extensive and enjoyable documentation of their round-the-world adventures.

The strong-livered teacher, flushed and vibrant, had carried them through, keeping herself and the children continuously refreshed with challenge. Together they had met the world, and it had met them. This method of progressing through the curriculum as travelogue, besides being highly stimulating to her preadolescent class, cleared away many of her own personal struggles with teaching what often seemed to her to be dull fundamentals.

RHYTHMIC RENEWAL

Heroines and heroes in many tales exemplify the liver's response to cries of distress. Modern knights-errant who have pledged their lives to the well-being of others embody its spirit. A fresh and healthy liver resembles a shield emblazoned splendidly with a blood-red cross. The Red Cross Knight in Edmund Spenser's seventeenth-century masterpiece *The Faerie Queen* willingly sets out to fulfill his high calling. Book One describes his battle with an enormously destructive dragon. Before the youthful and saintly knight (whose other name is Saint George) goes to battle, a holy hermit awakens within him a spiritual vision that strengthens his will for selfless service. Like many modern heroes, this knight battles the thrashing dark force assigned to him, and is almost destroyed by it. After the first exhausting day of battle, a stream bathes all his wounds with healing waters. During the second night, a tree refreshes his poisoned battle blood. When he rises, each time he is whole and strong, revived and refreshed. At the end of the story, the dragon is conquered and Saint George, perfected through his selfless deeds, shares his adventures with all the land, and with his most beloved.

Wherever you live on Earth, as the light lessens in the afternoon, you feel the liver's energies shift. As the liver's energies dip down with the Sun, a hunger for quick pick-me-ups can arise. The liver's clock, tuned to universal time and the movement of the Sun through the sky, finds deepest repose by midnight. Do you turn over, feeling restless, depressed, and hopeless, as liver activity awakens around three in the morning? Do you feel the same as it begins its twelve-hour cycle of rest around three in the afternoon? A main meal before three o'clock in the afternoon and a peaceful bowl of soup at the end of the day can bring comfort to the soul and ease you into a more refreshing night's sleep.

SHARING THE PROMETHEAN LEGACY

Stories tuned to the archetypal liver can help welcome relaxation. Storytelling can be healing medicine for those whose lives lack deep rest. In today's electronic world, multitudes are deprived of regenerative sleep. As we turn down the lights to a gentle glow and come into wise darkness, the embracing and ancient rhythmic world gently rocks and restores us. In monastic life, three to four o'clock in the morning is a natural time for waking gradually through prayer and meditation. From a good night's rest comes sparkling clarity and childlike joy. Healthy children often seem to levitate out of bed, streaming with life as they rush to meet the day.

The myth of Prometheus reflects the daily rhythmic drama of the liver. This ancient myth tells of giant Titans who made human beings out of themselves.

> At first the gods and these new men lived together, ate the same food, drank the same wine, and sang the same songs. But Zeus, the eldest god, did not like the new human beings. Prometheus, whose name means "foresight," felt compassion for the hu-

mans who were cold in winter with no roofs over their heads and no fires. Early one dawn, Prometheus concealed a ray of sunrise in the stalk of a green herb. In this way, he brought bright warmth for the first time into the newly created world of human beings. With the power of the Sun's rays, he taught them how to build earthly fires and to make tools for planting, harvesting, cooking, and building. Against the will of Zeus, the friendly god taught human beings the enjoyment of other arts.

Zeus awoke one day, irritated by all the points of light shining on Earth and threatening his power. He called Prometheus to atone for his willfulness by offering a sacrificial feast. Prometheus obeyed, but slyly. He slayed a bull and then hid the flesh. Then he smoothed the bones and sinew with glistening tempting fat and covered them with hide. The gods descended and chose to accept this offering. Only then did Zeus see that they had been tricked. The flesh went to the humans. Zeus was furious, so the myth goes, and commanded Prometheus to be chained with iron links to a craggy peak in the high Caucasus Mountains to assure he would not escape. Then Zeus thrust a stake through Prometheus' side. There he hung, day by day, blistered by the sun, beaten by the wind and rain. Zeus added to his suffering by sending a bird every morning to peck and tear at his liver. As light waned, the bird flew away, and each night within the mountainous depths of Prometheus's body, the liver majestically restored itself, only to be destroyed again the next day. This torture continued for countless years.

Many beings loved Prometheus and pleaded for his rescue, but he remained pinioned to that rock. At last, the great hero Hercules came along and took on his fate in willing service…but that is another story.

Prometheus gave humanity fire and the growing inner light of consciousness. In the mythical mountains of our bodies, he gave us the power of choice to live with abundant warmth and light. Many today are the sons and daughters of Prometheus, willing to suffer in order to serve the well-being and upliftment of others.

A venerable story from the Celtic tradition is also full of liver-rich imagery.

⊷⊷⊷⊷⊷

The Elucidation (or The Fisher King)

There is a world within this world, where once reigned a Fisher King. It is said that his lands were rich and fertile, with lush green meadows and bubbling brooks, streams, and wells. The people brought offerings to their springs and wells and decorated them with beautiful objects, so deep was their love and respect for those places. If you were wayfaring in that land, you would find a network of watering places, each one served by pure maidens who bore in their hands golden cups and whatever you desired for nourishment. The king protected these damsels.

But one day into that land rode a cruel king. He and his crude men were hot and hungry. They brought no offerings to the wells and they gave no thanks. The damsels came to them offering water from golden cups and asked them what it was they desired. But they had eyes only for what price the luminous cups would fetch at the markets. Their leader snatched a cup and threw a beautiful maiden on the ground and took his will of her. His men followed their master's example. And so they rode from spring to spring, from well to well, looting and abducting, until the forests were filled with weeping. The waters began to shrink and the trees became bare. Soon the land of plenty was nothing but a wasteland. The Fisher King lay wounded because each injury inflicted on the maidens he took upon himself. He and his court hid away from the eyes of men. From that time onward, all wayfarers in that land thirsted and hungered.

Time passed. At last there came another king called Arthur. The new king and his knights were trustworthy. They were hearty, full of good humor, will, and strength. When they heard what had happened, they vowed to replenish the land and rescue the maidens. That is how the Knights of the Round Table came to be, and how their great service to humanity began.

⚜⚜⚜⚜⚜

JORINDA AND JORINGEL REVISITED

A woman who attended one of my transformational storytelling courses had suffered much abuse in her childhood. She longed to be liberated from her past, and all the resentment and hurt she had felt over many years. During the course, as the group was reading "Jorinda and Joringel," a tale among those collected by the Grimm brothers, she decided to ignore her depression and honor her imagination. The tale portrays a sorceress who resented all lovers. You, too, like this woman, can take some time to focus on a dark character in a traditional fairy tale, then make a new story in which this character discovers positive feelings. To appreciate her story, first read the tale "Jorinda and Joringel."

The woman who attended the course wanted to know whether the hag in the story had been born wicked and cruel. She slipped away from the class to write an expanded version of the fairy tale. Later, she returned, amazed by the flowing clarity of her imagination. She had written a story that had the effect of a powerful healing dream. Her story was about a princess who was brought up by servants in a cold gray room.

No fire was allowed in the fireplace. Each of her suitors was cruelly banished by her father, the king. Her only pleasures were to see birds flying past a narrow stone window and to listen to their beautiful songs.

After the king died, his ghost haunted the castle the princess had inherited from him, threatening her every step. In her loneliness, she sent her servants out with wicker baskets in search of birds. Each morning she would cry, "Bring more birds! I must have more birds!"

Finally, one day, the servants could find no more birds. The princess became very angry. She beat the servants and drove them from the castle. Then she went into the forest to search for birds herself.

As years passed, the princess's resentment increased, especially toward fair young maidens who were not imprisoned as she had been in her youth. One day as she wandered disconsolately through the castle, she happened upon some musty old books. In them she found a spell to change maidens into birds. After that, whenever young lovers came close to the castle, she spat black bile and harassed them in the form of an owl until she had captured the girls. When Jorinda and her beloved Joringel wandered too close to her realm, Jorinda, too, met this fate, and had to live in a dark cage as a disembodied bird with the others.

But at last, Jorinda's lover brought a magic flower, red as healthy fresh blood, to the castle. Under the protection of this flower, the princess could do no harm to Joringel, and so he was able to enter the castle, open the cages, and liberate his beloved Jorinda and all the other maidens. Seeing them set free, the sorceress princess wept as she had never wept before. She wept so long on the cold stone floor that she became ill.

The woman's story continued with power that astonished her and the listening group:

Now it happened that in former years, one of the castle servants had been secretly in love with the princess. He had been sorry to see her imprisoned through her youth. A humble youth, he had never ventured to speak of his love. When the princess turned all her servants out of the castle, he had wandered the world. At last he decided to return to the castle, ready to serve the princess in any way.

He arrived just at the time of her fit of weeping and utter emotional exhaustion. Lifting the princess from the stone floor, he placed her on a couch with a warm cover. Soon he lit a fire in the bleak hearth. The princess was ill, with a deathly green hue to her skin. As the servant worked, the princess babbled deliriously in her fever about a "magic red flower."

She continued to be ill for many days, and once while she was sleeping, the servant quietly left the castle and inquired about Jorinda and Joringel. When at last he found them, he told them everything about the princess's hard childhood.

Joringel said to the servant: "Since it is a magic flower, it would not be right to keep it entirely to ourselves when another has need."

And so the servant set off for the castle with the red flower, and new hope.

"Dear Princess, is it too late?" the devoted servant asked sadly. He touched the red flower to her ashen cheeks.

Slowly, the slightest pink came into her face. She opened her eyes.

Gradually, the princess regained her strength and began to flush with happiness in their friendship. Feeling open and alive together, they decided to make the castle a place of beauty. They planted gardens. In time, the villagers overcame their fear and came to the castle often for feasting and dancing. Jorinda and Joringel came with them. The halls echoed with the sounds of children running, laughing, and playing to the music of freely winging birds.

The student's face glowed as she exclaimed, "Here was an assignment I could do! I know story writing is not a cure-all, but as I wrote this story I had a deep feeling of truth. The flower represents a healthy fresh flow of blood within my own liver. Then compassion poured through me like clear water. I began resonating with moral principles. Morality filled the plot and my choice of words. Later I could relate more clearly to the witch elements when I felt grim and isolated in myself. I saw how I sometimes draw rejection to myself. The story helps me to accept and work on myself, and to really enjoy my life!"

Transformational Storytelling

Liver Affirmation

As I will to serve others, I am restored to life.

Basic Liver Story Dynamic

Emotionality matures into selfless service.

Liver Protagonists and Antagonists

Liver protagonists (characters who support liver health) devote themselves to freedom and liberation. They are willing to be leaned on, and are eager for adventure and travel. They love to laugh, yet are sensitive to the needs and desires of others.

Liver antagonists (characters who express liver dysfunction) are irritable, resentful, hostile, and hypochondriacal. In codependent tangles, they prohibit and repress desires and feelings. They laugh too loudly and too long, spewing emotions and words without respect for others or themselves.

Basic Story Elements

Myths and stories often resonate with specific internal processes. This reliable pattern invokes well-being and resilience in every cell of your body:

Setting Out: The protagonist sets out in quest of greater love, strength, justice, wisdom, and happiness.

Trouble: One or more obstacles and/or antagonists interfere with the journey.

Help: Wise and benevolent help comes, often giving a gift.

Positive Ending: The protagonist fulfils the quest with joy and celebration.

SUMMONING YOUR STORYTELLER

Liver-strong storytellers feel eager to embark on adventures as they share emotionally charged stories. Their voices tend to be buoyant and their words exuberant. Their gestures express a wide range of feelings. Their colorful outfits display the inner excitement they feel. Keenly attuned to the emotional responsiveness of their audiences, they ride with their characters on uplifting waves of emotion. They especially admire the sort of storyteller of whom it is said: "There is not a dry eye when she tells a story." Whether crying from laughter or sorrow, they enter into their stories with bubbling and infectious enthusiasm.

Exercises to Explore and Balance the Liver

The life and times of your liver. Like most people, do you long for more restorative peace and sleep? Attuning to the natural rhythms of the liver is challenging on our twenty-four-hour supermarket superhighways, yet everyone's blood sugar level still rises naturally to meet each new dawn. Do you wake early feeling eager for life? Like Marit Jarstad recovering from hepatitis B, take time to commune with your liver. How did it serve your life today? What emotional and food battles has it recently fought for you? Write the autobiographical adventures of your liver today. Cast whatever toxins you are aware of into imaginative pictures.

Rehearsing for a grand journey. De-*livering* freely expressed emotion can be a gift to others. Imagine you are arousing enthusiasm in two or three of your best friends for going on a wonderful journey together. Breathe generously. Place a hand on your lower ribs and gently shake your liver up and down, back and forth, until you feel warm laughter rising. Then with a ruby-rich exuberant voice imagine yourself telling your friends what they have to look forward to on this journey.

Dance with Jupiter. Music and dance stir imagination. To invite a liver story to arise spontaneously, listen to the opening movement of Mozart's *Jupiter* Symphony or Beethoven's Seventh Symphony. In ancient Greek medical lore, the liver was connected with Jupiter, and for good reasons. As you listen to the symphony, alone or with a partner, enact a liver battle. Take turns embodying a toxic invader and a healthy liver. Dance freshly oxygenated, iron-rich blood surging through the liver after eating, for example, a fresh spinach salad. For contrast, portray the liver struggling to transform a heavy fatty meal.

Transform toxicity. Where health is suppressed, imagination can arise to put things right. Your physical and emotional bodies are closely connected. Describe a toxic force in your life, perhaps the influence of another person, or something in your environment that has a negative effect on you.

Now tell an imaginative adventure story about a hero or heroine who sets off with effervescent laughter in a magical flying ship to cleanse a landscape of toxicity. Along the way, gather all the helpers needed to accomplish this great task.

The gallbladder often constricts the vocal cords, but the liver can cause the voice to gush with a rich emotion. Unfurl your words like ferns in a lush woodland.

Protagonist meets antagonist. Set a clock for twenty minutes. On a large piece of unlined paper, with brightly colored pencils or ink, write a story in which the virtues and the shadows of the liver confront each other. Let the protagonist move with determination toward a positive ending.

Colorful emotions. Sit with colored crayons and, through the colors you use, portray one by one the emotions that unfold in a story you love. Bring out those same colors in your voice as you tell the story. Two calls to wakefulness were inscribed over the portals of the temple at Delphi: "Nothing in excess" and "Know thyself." Storytellers who freely express emotions rather than portraying them in words can deprive their listeners of freedom to feel emotions for themselves.

The power of selfless service. Describe a selfless servant who will not abandon someone in great distress, or who comes to set a whole people free. Describe this knight or warrioress, modern firefighter, or roving reporter who is "liverish," feeling irritable, perhaps eating and drinking too much. Yet when called to high duty, your protagonist swings into glorious action. Who is saved by this hero's willing deeds?

Describe someone you know who is a modern son or daughter of Saint George in the world today. Perhaps it is yourself.

EXPANDING LIVER AWARENESS THROUGH DANCE, MUSIC, AND YOGA

Dance

Plant your feet firmly and with your elbows close at your sides, breathe a grand breath of bubbling joy as you rub your liver, making small circles with your hand. Move your whole torso in small and larger circles from left to right. Then gradually lift your arms above your head as you bend and sway in every direction, like a great tree or a whole forest in a moist warm wind. Imagine you are drawing people upward and onward with you for a good cause.

Music
Mozart, *Jupiter* Symphony no. 41, the third movement
Smetana, *The Moldau*
Schubert, *The Trout Quintet*

Yoga asanas (Sanskrit names in italics)
Standing Crescent Moon *(Ardha Chandrasana)*
Abdominal Twist *(Jathara Parivrtti)*
Reclining Hand to Big Toe *(Septa Padangusthasana)*

4

Decision-Maker: The Gallbladder

"**Y**ou have a lot of gall!" we exclaim with admiration, and sometimes a twinge of distaste. The pear-shaped gall sack is tucked neatly just under the right lobe of the liver. Its bitter yellow gall fluid is continuously produced by surpluses in the liver. Ever ready for action, through its exact sensing of the needs of the digestive system, it is a little stove that efficiently stashes away bile to convert fat into energy. As it supports and assists digestion, the gallbladder can very quickly fire up and distribute sparkle to the whole house of the body, adding dash to both the personality and the digestive system.

The hot and complex relationship of the gallbladder with the body and psyche differs from warmth of heart and from sexual fire. The gallbladder generates brave fiery thoughts, the nerve to act on them and to follow through. It identifies the "fat" of confused excesses at the physiological level and goes to work. Like e-mails firing up millions of people to address important issues, gall generates decisive action within the body, as well as in families and in places of learning, business, and government. Gall-strong people have a natural cleansing effect on others. They generate dashing life stories.

Try tracing on your own body the zigzag of the gallbladder meridian from head to toe. This energy line activates the dynamics of resistance throughout the body. Without contraries, there is no progression; especially through the work of the gallbladder, we experience that every impulse sets into motion an equal and opposite force. The energy of the gallbladder meridian first pushes back from the outer corner of each eye, one branch weaving a vigorous pathway to and fro across

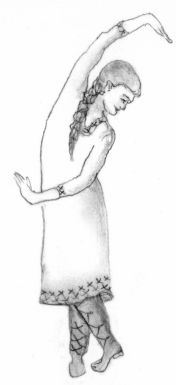

Gallbladder Exercise

the head, before it plummets to the shoulders and rib cage and then the hips. Another energy line crosses the cheeks and moves internally through the neck and chest to the gallbladder itself. From there this line connects in the hip with the other branch and descends along the outer thighs and knees to its releasing place on the inside tip of the fourth toe. It also branches over with heated verve to the big toes and eventually greets the liver lines where they begin their ascent.

The gallbladder meridian helps to fire up digestion and assimilation throughout the body. According to traditional Chinese medicine, it builds and nourishes the tendons that weave together bone and muscle. To feel gall energy gathering within yourself, straighten your back. With your feet firmly on the floor, pressing down with your big toes, bend down and press your fingers on the gall points located on the outside of your legs midway down the calves. Stand up again, relax your belly, and breathe in and out of your whole torso, until you feel your body heating up. Then stand and firmly scissor your hands above your head, right wrist over left, left over right, as you take in and release a series of swift full-body breaths.

GALLBLADDER AND LIVER BALANCE WITHIN THE BODY AND PSYCHE

Through what long eons has this relationship evolved? When the responsive and intuitive liver generates distress signals, gall with its crisscrossing energies quickly rises and knits a "thinking cap." It helps us to use logic to forge successful strategies, make decisions, and construct boundaries. If we grow weak and watery with emotion, the gallbladder can fire up sudden boundaries and blazing resolves. If we lose our way, the volatile little fire pit of the gallbladder sends emergency signals to the brain, as

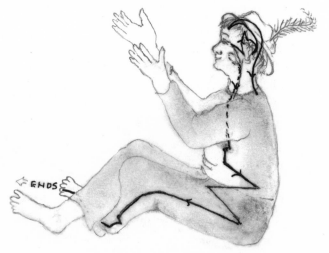

The Gallbladder Meridian

together brain and gallbladder instigate practical step-by-step planning that in emergency situations will override the consensus of the rest of the body. It incites a restless drive to sort and deal with contradictory voices. You may know this voice in yourself, the one that loves debate and always manages to find a different point of view.

Bile activity, intensified by the gallbladder, stimulates "eager beaver" choices. People with strong gall activity are especially gifted in crises. Their quick scissor-sharp decisions often rule in emergency situations. As relief for fret and anguish, many organizations hire gall-strong experts who assist bogged-down bureaucracies in sorting out problems and negotiating changes. Bile activity also supports exhilarating winning tactics in courtrooms and in golf and tennis tournaments. It bestows additional skill on the surgeon's scalpel. Gall-informed intelligence helps people reduce congestion in busy intersections with traffic signals and control towers; it is at work in efficient line managers and job foremen. Gall activity supports acupuncturists and well-organized teachers, and all those who follow through from A to Z to untangle problems, whether medical, legal, mathematical, political, or in community service. It helps in the invention of such useful devices as pulleys and windshield wipers. Enlisting the help of the brain and nurturing a sense of responsibility, the gallbladder fires along editing procedures, grammar rules, and library systems. It shapes protocols for ballroom dancing and skating competitions, diagrams for knitting, and directions for organizing kitchen or shop.

A twelve-year-old, inspired by his own lively gall process, decided to travel each of the twelve major bus routes in his city. After he had studied the efficiency of each one, he sent in a proposal for practical improvements to the county council. He was later invited to share his well thought-out presentations with the council, which implemented a number of his suggestions.

A restaurant owner with a dashing abundance of gall insists, "Life is all about choices!" He enjoys watching people face the tasty array on his menus. "Each morning," he says, "I wake up and say to myself, 'I can choose to be in a good mood or to be in a bad mood.' I always choose to be in a good mood. Each time something bad happens, I can choose to be a victim or to learn from it. I always choose to learn. I choose the positive side of life." His philosophy is: "It's your choice how you live your life."

The Gall's Momentum and Timing

When I took a journey with a gall-strong friend, Maggie's behavior resembled the gallbladder studying a fatty meal so that it can be absorbed and heat up the whole body as efficiently and smoothly as possible. She had mapped every detail of the journey in advance, securing the itinerary to a clipboard so it would be easy to read while we were on the road. Thinking ahead with care to every need, she devotedly and efficiently organized the car. Once we started out, she preferred to travel in the fast lane. "I like to leave late, and go fast," she said. When she wasn't driving, she studied signs diligently, jotting down details to improve the return route. At each crossroad, she heatedly pointed out the right direction with her whole arm, sometimes with both arms, like a pair of tailor's scissors.

"I tend to approach life from my hot little head," says Maggie, as she struggles with daily bursts of Promethean ardor. "This sometimes makes me very uncomfortable to live with. Give me a messy room and I clean and put it right into order! Whenever a mistake is made, a huge drive arises within me to prevent it from happening ever again."

A man with a similar pattern says, "It feels like my gallbladder inflates like a sausage stuffed with work and worry, and no enjoyment. It's an understatement to say that I am unable to relax. When I am fired up about a project, I have a relentless drive to accomplish it well to completion. I push myself at a relentless pace, and then I inevitably drop."

Stressed gall energy tends to create high-pressured headaches as the bile works to balance digestive forces. It is not surprising that gall-strong people sometimes collapse with migraine headaches and go in search of healers. Maggie explains, "I semiconsciously create extremes, rather than endure phlegmatic humdrum. When I attract dramatic excitement and variety, it usually backfires and turns into disorder and chaos!" Who hasn't felt under fire by those who want to reorganize your life, or zealously challenge your thinking? "When I am under pressure," Maggie says, "my compulsive organizing tends to 'go haywire' and I have to collapse into complete and painful rest. Every night in my sleep I feel as though I am accumulating unidentifiable toxins during the night. On waking, I sometimes feel so ill, I don't want to stay in my body a single instant more. I throw up and cannot eat or drink. My nerves are raw as my gall spurts strangely in response to food. It invades my stomach and has to come up."

"But after a migraine," she adds cheerfully, "I feel cleansed, energized, and ready for action. I go from the gates of hell, to clarity."

TIME OUT OF MIND

When Maggie was vigorously battling a series of headaches, she decided to experiment with storytelling as a healing art. Typically, the gallbladder waits, fires, and then rapidly restores itself. As she worked with its rhythms, she was often trying to catch up with herself in intensive bouts and struggling to be on time. "It is a cycle," she explained. "I am always catching up from the things I couldn't get done yesterday, so I do double time today, which leads to another migraine." She was bothered by a recurring nightmare in which she had twenty minutes to get to Italy, and her bags were not packed. Maggie created a story in response to this dream that gave her new perspective on her pressured headaches and compulsion to immediate action. The main character of her story was a princess, who was constantly arguing with Time.

The Princess Who Longed for Time

In the morning when the castle bells chimed, a princess slept on in the clock tower. When she arrived late for breakfast, the king was grumpy and the queen fired many a cook. At length, the king and queen sent the princess away to another castle. Ordinary time did not exist in her new abode and there she arose when she wished. There she lived for a while and did as she pleased. She ate breakfast at midnight if she chose, and arose after noon if she wished. Eventually, however, the Princess began to long for time. At long last, she journeyed home to find that a full two hundred years had gone by, and that the castle was now a shopping mall. She bought a watch in the mall, an alarm clock, and a wall clock, and rented an apartment above the watch repair shop. She set all her clocks and went out to the café to show the people her new timepiece and her new up-to-date clothes, and to begin a new life....

CHOICES IN STORIES

Hephaestus, the Greek god whose task is to work at a fiery forge, is a vivid mythic version of the gall fire at work. With hammer and tongs, this mighty son of Zeus heats metals and beats out firm tools for the survival tactics of gods and men. From a traditional planetary perspective, Mars rules gall with a will of iron, helping us stand our ground, form words, and speak. Yet often choice is not a simple matter. As it burns up fears, gall activity tends to stimulate ardent morality with an attorney's energy. A Cherokee spoke to his grandson about a battle that was going on inside him:

Two Wolves

"My son," he said, "life is lived between two wolves. One is full of anger, envy, sorrow, self-pity, inferiority, and superiority. The other is full of joy, peace, hope, humility, kindness, and faith."

The grandson asked his grandfather, "Which wolf wins?"

The old man simply replied, "The one I feed."

Stephen Vincent Benét's tale "The Devil and Daniel Webster" shows both sides of gall in action in the struggle of Daniel Webster for inner clarity.

Jabez Stone, a farmer whose luck has turned, said in his desperation, "I vow it's enough to make a man want to sell his soul to the devil!" The devil soon appeared to him and they struck a seven-year bargain. After that, Jabez Stone began to prosper. His land and cattle thrived. Lightning that struck all over his valley would jump over his barn. When Jabez Stone's deal with the devil was almost up, "sick with terror," he sought out Daniel Webster, the greatest attorney in America. Daniel walked up and down as he listened to both parties with fiery intensity, hands behind his back, now and then asking a question, or turning his eyes to the floor, "as if they'd bore through it like gimlets." When Jabez Stone had finished and the devil approached his client, Webster stood his ground. A jury was summoned. Webster's veins stood out on his forehead, but through every opposing argument his voice remained clear.

"Dan'l began to heat, like an iron in the forge. When he got up to speak, he was going to flay that stranger with every trick known to the law, and the judge and jury too. He didn't care if it was contempt of court or what would happen to him.... He just got madder and madder, thinking of what he'd say.

"Then this great man saw as clear as day that it was his own anger and horror burning in the eyes of the opposition, and he knew he would have to wipe it out of himself. He stood there for a moment, his black eyes burning like anthracite. And then he began to speak. He started off in a low voice, though you could hear every word. They say he could call on the harps of the blessed when he chose. He didn't start out by condemning or reviling. He was precisely speaking about the things that make a country a country, a man a man."

The tale ends: "The devil gives a wide berth to that territory ever since." When such a capacity for decisive, fiery power is held back, it is not surprising that gall-strong people experience throat tensions and a cramped and even desperate need to ease themselves through talk.

Balancing Gall's Energies

Almost everyone experiences at times unpleasant bloating and burping, or pain along the gallbladder meridian lines as gallstones and other debris block the gallbladder ducts. When the bile duct becomes overloaded with cholesterol, body and soul no longer feel so keenly the power of decision. A gallbladder that is not functioning to its fullest potential can create vexations in both body and soul. Just as a clogged gallbladder can affect thoughts and feelings, in a reciprocal action, negative emotions can aggravate the gallbladder. Is it any wonder that so many gallbladders are removed every day? Many of us are adept at surrounding ourselves in fears, and at storing worries and anxieties, especially fear of mistakes or failure. "Yes, but..." habits of mind can paralyze confidence. Timidity and fear are signs of weakened gall activity, just as pressured rash decisions can result from excess gall.

Yet as health is restored, the gallbladder continues to fire up the energy of self-esteem. Even if a gallbladder has been physically removed, gall strength continues to work in the total energy field of the body. It thrives as we meet challenges, questions and answers, riddles and wit. Just as gall waits to be ignited into action, well-balanced, gall-strong people seek the flint and tinder of tests wherever they go. They learn to endure the friction of confrontation, using their thoughts and words to face challenges. Gall-strong people, like Daniel Webster, jump in. Like Daniel's, their words can be as effective as those of a wizard who is sitting, as Benét wrote in his masterpiece of a story, "like a glowing coal, weaving a spell to dispel the plague."

A famous Viennese physician, speaking to his students, said, "A surgeon needs two gifts: the power of observation and freedom from nausea." He then dipped his fourth finger into some repulsive fluid and licked it, requesting each of the students to do the same. They steeled themselves and managed as best they could to imitate him without flinching. With a smile, the surgeon then said, "Gentlemen, I congratulate you on having passed the first test. But not, unfortunately, the second. For not one of you noticed that the finger I licked was not the one I dipped into the fluid."

A very old story, the forerunner to Shakespeare's play *The Merchant of Venice,* exemplifies both unbalanced and balanced gall activity. It tells of the son of a prominent merchant who lost a desperate bargain.

> As the youth sat praying to be saved from having a pound of his flesh cut from his body, a king's daughter noticed him. Having "gall" and a quick and clever mind, she disguised herself as a lawyer and defended the youth, saying with characteristic precision, "I insist that exactly one kilogram of this man's flesh be cut in a single stroke." The merchant realized that, as a result of his bargain, the young man would die. Then the king's daughter, still in her disguise, said, "Perhaps there is a way to provide justice and kindness. Let the merchant receive the labor of the young man until the debt is paid. The young man needs a mentor. The merchant needs to temper his ethics with concern for more than money. All will gain from such a result." Hearing this sage advice so brilliantly put forth, the young man was saved, and the king invited his daughter to sit at his right hand and guide him for the rest of his days.

Healthy balanced gall inspires a sensible way forward for everyone. It strides with sure steps and diligent logical thinking toward the sphinx posing life or death riddles. It teaches important lessons with trickster ingenuity, sometimes with a smile and a wink, as in this humorous story-poem by Ogden Nash:

The Adventures of Isabel

Isabel met an enormous bear,
Isabel, Isabel didn't care;
The bear was hungry, the bear was ravenous,
The bear's big mouth was cruel and cavernous.
The bear said, Isabel, glad to meet you,
How do, Isabel, now I'll eat you!
Isabel, Isabel, didn't worry,
Isabel didn't scream or scurry.
She washed her hands and she straightened her hair up,
Then Isabel quietly ate the bear up.

Once in a night as black as pitch
Isabel met a wicked old witch.
The witch's face was cross and wrinkled,
The witch's gums with teeth were sprinkled.
Ho ho, Isabel! the old witch crowed,
I'll turn you into an ugly toad!
Isabel, Isabel, didn't worry,
Isabel didn't scream or scurry,
She showed no rage and she showed no rancour,
But she turned the witch into milk and drank her.

Isabel met a hideous giant,
Isabel continued self-reliant.
The giant was hairy, the giant was horrid,
He had one eye in the middle of his forehead.
Good morning, Isabel, the giant said,
I'll grind your bones to make my bread.
Isabel, Isabel, didn't worry,
Isabel didn't scream or scurry.
She nibbled the zwieback that she always fed off,
And when it was gone, she cut the giant's head off.

Isabel met a troublesome doctor,
He punched and he poked till he really shocked her.
The doctor's talk was of coughs and chills

And the doctor's satchel bulged with pills.
The doctor said unto Isabel,
Swallow this, it will make you well.
Isabel, Isabel, didn't worry,
Isabel didn't scream or scurry.
She took those pills from the pill concocter,
And Isabel calmly cured the doctor.

⋆⋇⋆⋇⋆⋇⋆

A woman of plentiful gall wisdom confided, "In emergencies, I always feel my smart edge protecting me and others." A rousing tale from Iraq also portrays clear thinking and a healthy supply of gall. As the story begins, Mohamed bin Bathera, a great king, has returned to his palace from war to discover that his wife has been unfaithful.

His rage is so great that, on pain of death, he banishes all women from his land except his mother. His decision is absolute, and no woman or girl dares to return to the kingdom until a bold young woman, out of curiosity and a sense of indignity, ventures over his border. Like the heroine in the Grimms' tale "The Twelve Huntsmen" who finds herself in similar circumstances, Sherifa disguises herself as a prince. This prince is soon ushered with great magnificence into the presence of the king. The king is puzzled because he feels such friendship and love for her. Sherifa faces three tests set by the king. With heated presence of mind, she chooses swords over silks and jewels, a meal of hot peppers over milder dishes, and ignores a crying child. She then rides at full gallop into the sea, rather than remove her clothes and be seen as a woman, and escapes, quickly hoisting sails for home. But she paused during her dash to the sea to write a fiery challenge above the door of the city:

Woman I came, I went no other,
To your despite, Hamed bin Bathera.

Seeing these words, the king defies anyone to stop him until he finds Sherifa. His search takes him far and wide. When at last he comes, dagger in hand, into her bedchamber, he finds her standing waiting for him, gloriously naked.

"You must answer my question before you kill me," she says.

Hamed replies, "What is your question?"

Then Sherifa, with perfect gall, asks, "What is a dagger without a sheath?"

The king replies, "A dagger without a sheath cannot be, for the blade would rust and decay."

With that, the Princess Sherifa says, "If there can be man without woman, then there can be a dagger without a sheath, for man is a sword blade and woman is a sheath that protects man, cooks his food, keeps his house, and fulfills his desires."

And so the king, filled with exceeding love for her, "turns his dagger to its sheath." Their reign together begins, and very soon girls and wives are returned in celebration to their realm.

Gall-strong people insist that life goes well. "Now" is an important word to them. They are determined not to collapse with mistakes, but instead to go freely about their tasks with devotion and workaholic determination, even if they must disappear for a time to pull themselves back from burnout. They want everyone to go ahead, ignoring fear, correcting themselves, even improving pronunciation or grammar in the midst of a dire emergency.

Transformational Storytelling
Gallbladder Affirmation
I transform what interferes with life.

Basic Gallbladder Story Dynamic
Uncertainty transforms into devoted decisive action.

Gallbladder Protagonists and Antagonists
Gallbladder protagonists (characters who support gallbladder health) are decisive and resolute. They possess chutzpah and pizzazz. As their strong will rises to their heads, they are dependable, committed, dutiful, and devoted to the well-being of all. They are bold in selfless service.

Gallbladder antagonists (characters who express gallbladder dysfunction) are cowardly, indecisive, devastated by loss or disappointment, and accusing of others. They tend to operate in the shadows, be secretive and hateful, and are their own worst enemies.

> ### Basic Story Elements
> Myths and stories often resonate with specific internal processes. This reliable pattern invokes well-being and resilience in every cell of your body:
>
> *Setting Out:* The protagonist sets out in quest of greater love, strength, justice, wisdom, and happiness.
>
> *Trouble:* One or more obstacles and/or antagonists interfere with the journey.
>
> *Help:* Wise and benevolent help comes, often giving a gift.
>
> *Positive Ending:* The protagonist fulfils the quest with joy and celebration.

Summoning Your Storyteller
With their propensity to argue and convince, fiery, gall-strong storytellers aim to tell stories that clear up muddled situations. They place their best foot forward, with vigorous will to cut through and sort out chaotic situations. Eyes alert and discerning, their angular forceful gestures

support the points they want to make. The stories they choose are grounded in practical realities. They hope their stories will help fire their listeners into action to bring about change. Their voices may ring sharply. Nothing wishy-washy in clothing or thoughts distracts them from their goal to forge tools to bring about clarity and improve life.

Exercises to Explore and Balance the Gallbladder

Going to the forge: an imaginative journey. Imagine visiting the crackling fiery forge of the great god Hephaestus as he makes tools for human beings and gods. His fire blazes and flares with smoke and incense. Ask this blacksmith to forge a useful tool to help you change a stressful situation in your life.

Create a brief story in which a gall-strong protagonist successfully outwits a dysfunctional antagonist, or becomes chief navigator and saves an expedition from disaster, or transforms an overgrown garden into a well-organized paradise.

Have a worry! The Persian poet Hafiz wrote, "Now that your worries have proven so un-lucrative, why not get yourself a better job?" How many of your worries can you list in seven minutes? Estimate how much energy you fire up to maintain these worries. Discern which ones are really useful to you. Now write the others on kindling wood or paper and set them alight; compost the ash.

Tuning the voice. A woman with chronic headaches decided to train herself to be more forth-right. Speaking clear, vigorous stories for children at a local library helped reduce her head-aches. She decided to train adults to tell stories with positive outcomes. Now she stands her own ground. She places a small square of carpet on the floor to help others to stand and speak clearly. The gallbladder strengthens will and the power of speech. Everyone needs to hear well-spoken words. Weak gall activity results in amorphous thought and words that wobble and fade into one another. Every word, phrase, and sentence has a beginning, middle, and end. Words can stream as healthy bile does into the digestive tract to act on fears and stagnant concepts and conditions, and to help us thrive.

Daniel Webster eloquently outwitted the devil. Describe an incident in your own life when heated gall activity supported you as you confronted opposition. Fire the power of positive en-ergy into each word you speak.

Decision now! Describe someone struggling with a decision, pondering different options, perhaps for years, despairing and confused. A man wrote the following indignant letter to his col-leagues during a challenging time at work: "Please clean up and reorganize this place from the top down!" Describe the firing up of both your body and your mind to make a decision. Gall-strong folk often see three or four possibilities. "That didn't work?" Quickly knocking on the next door, they say, "Let's try another way."

Putting things right. What in your life do you want to put right? Call on gallbladder energy to organize and map a time frame to accomplish this project. Write down a sequence of steps for achieving your goal, and list and number the resources you need. After you have laid out your plans, share them with a partner. Ask a willing listener to advise you on how to accomplish your project more effectively.

Solving big problems. Read the inspiring children's book by Demi, *One Grain of Rice.* This tale tells about the skillful transformation of a very large social problem. Retell this story with the strong will and exactitude that characterizes gall-strong energies.

Your traveling style. Describe yourself getting ready to take a journey. How do you prepare? Do you make checklists, gather maps, book in advance? Would you like more procedure and thoroughness? If you were traveling around the world, would you prefer to wander impromptu, or to have a clearly organized itinerary?

Seeking to balance gall and liver energies. A woman who felt the intensity of her gall at an early age remembered her liver-strong grandmother. "Grandma would sit mending while she told me stories about an imaginary boat in our backyard. In it we would visit all our friends and neighbors." Gall and liver energies balance one another. To bring ballast to the persistent intensities of the gallbladder, create a storyteller who is round and soft, and full of liver-rich warmth and imagination.

The liver and gallbladder are needed more than ever today to bring resourceful consciousness to our environmental challenges. Everywhere, heroic deeds, large and small, call us to cheerful, willing activity. Bring both gall and liver energies together to change something in your family or community with warmth, decision, and complete effectiveness.

EXPANDING GALLBLADDER AWARENESS THROUGH DANCE, MUSIC, AND YOGA

Dance
Vigorously crisscross your right and left arms, hands, and, one at a time, your fingers, while at the same time crisscrossing your feet and your legs. This dance can also be done seated in a chair.

Music
Prokofiev, *Classical Symphony*
Franz Liszt, Hungarian Rhapsody no. 12 in C-sharp Minor and no. 6 in D-flat

Yoga asanas (Sanskrit names in italics)
Standing and seated leg cradling *(Yoga mudrasana)*
Cowfaced Pose of Nobility *(Gomukhasana)*
Pigeon *(Ekha Pada Rajakapotasana)*

5

Perfecting Spirit: The Large Intestine

From ileum to anus, the large intestine forms a sensitive undulating archway enfolding the smoother convolutions of the small intestine. Trillions of bacteria housed within these final five feet of the intestinal tract help it to produce vitamins and minerals. When these are excreted, they release subtle constructive and refining energies to the body, and to the earth. Your large intestinal tract is like a compost pile in the garden of your body, and like a miner's lode in its cavernous depths. It forms and stores vitamins and minerals in a way similar to the formation of gems and metals in the mineral-rich earth. As our bodies draw these subtle forces into larger circulation, we glow sometimes with exquisite luster as their luminosities nourish us in both body and soul.

To experience the slowly pulsing digestive rhythms of your large intestinal tract, sit and press your outstretched hands, especially your pointer fingers, against your thighs. Straighten your back, push down with your heels, breathe deeply a few times, and then relax completely. To feel the warm pulsations of your transverse colon, place your hand just below your rib cage and rub your belly from right to left, following the natural direction of colonic flow. Another way to increase the rhythmic digestive activity in your large intestine is to cross one arm over the other at the elbow. Then try to press your palms together. Similarly, try crossing the knee opposite to the crossing arm over the other leg, linking your foot under the calf. Breathe and rhythmically contract and release the now opposing and intertwining arms and legs. Grip vigorously, engaging all your muscles, and breathe in and out several times. Then reverse sides. In these pretzel positions, the twined arms and legs resemble the undulating muscularity of the lower bowel.

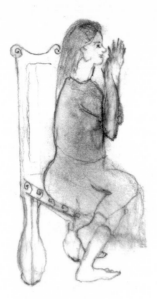

Large Intestine Exercise

In the Chinese medical view of the body, the extensive energy line of the large intestine begins at the tip of the index finger and moves upward along the thumb and forearm to the elbow and the upper arm. At a sensitive point in the shoulder, it divides, one branch flowing downward through the lung and diaphragm into the ascending colon. The other branch rises through the neck into the lower jaw to nourish our gums and teeth, crosses over, and exits beside the nose on the opposite side of the face.

In Search of a Glowing Rhythmic Flow

A healthy human large intestine cooperates vigorously with ecological necessity. When I was a young teacher in England I lived on a wonderful farm. During the winter months, we would ply our Jersey cows with hay and great bunches of dried herbs to add flavor and substance to the milk for the children. Around the barn, the odor of cow dung was sweet and strong. By early spring, it had matured to a rich odorless perfection. As the farmhands turned it into the gardens by hand, our nostrils filled up with its potent magic. In our more human world, "restrooms" tend to sanitize away such exhilarating activities. As it provides the last chance for the body to make something out of the food in our digestive system, the grand finale mood of the large intestine has a life of its own. Stinky at times, its elegance nevertheless contributes more to our well-being than we may realize. In fact, all cells enjoy and sometimes struggle with the rhythms of excretion.

Like any part of us, the large intestine as it monitors the final stages of digestive enterprise can pleasantly relax and flow, or seize up and "go to pieces." People in rural, nonindustrialized areas who live simple natural lives under little stress beam brightly and squat after every major meal, as the bowel moves its contents thoroughly in a smooth undulation. All bodily organs depend on the rhythmic health of the large intestine. Yet fecal "waste" in our stressful lives can too often rush out too quickly for its nutrients to

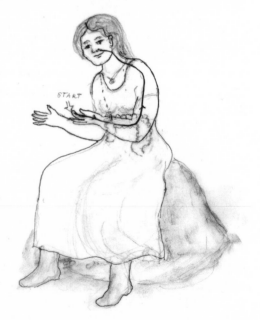

The Large Intestine Meridian

be absorbed, exhausting both body and soul. As a result, our thoughts and speech can also become diarrhetic. Attempts at conversation can become amorphous and out of touch with the thoughts or feelings of others. Intestinal struggles can also compact and back up within us for long periods of time, resulting in pressured, lethargic resistance of body and soul. During these sluggish times, we feel grumpy, stubborn, and out of control. The skin dulls and overtaxed digestion raises bumps. This is why cleansing the bowel with many glasses of water, salts, herbs, and enemas is a standard cure throughout the world for a load of problems. As we shall see, storytelling, too, can help the large intestine come into balance.

DISCOVERING COMPOST TREASURE

Necessary minerals and other substances compacted in the many interstices of the large intestinal wall can be stored there for many months or even years before they are released into the bloodstream to strengthen the body. The opening story in Heinrich Zimmer's famous collection called *The King and the Corpse* portrays in picture language the exquisite transformative mysteries hidden in the large intestine. It tells of a king who was visited every day by a holy man. The holy man would silently offer him a piece of fruit. The king would accept the gift and toss it into his treasure house. After a time, there lay a mass of fruit in various stages of decay and, amidst the debris, a heap of priceless gems. That was the beginning of the king's discovery of the inestimable physical, mental and spiritual value of compost.

Those who healthily inhabit the realm of the large intestine tend to be solidly built, with strong muscles in torso and limbs, and sturdy glowing faces. Whether hefty or slender, their internal world is rich, large, and full of organizing activity. As the meticulous discernment of the large intestine is reflected in their personalities, they can be unusually caring and constructive. They tend to bring out the richesse in everyone they know, and are usually reasonable and tolerant. They love to see the absolute best potential in others and to support that. As detailed work unfolds, they seek perfection in every detail, and bring balance through attending to overview as well as to details. They try hard to improve and enrich the world outside them, and to inspire others toward ambitious and worthy goals. This striving for them can be a tremendous joy. The constant inner longing for beautiful results showers them in a transcendent glow. Powerful gripping life forces in the gut lining release stunning mineral luminosities. A clear jeweled brightness gleams through their skin and their whole demeanor.

As jewelers within the general psyche of human beings, these people gain inner strength in applying their perfecting genius to constructive activities. Their self-confidence comes from subordinating themselves to an ideal and striving toward perfection, determined every day to make their ideals a reality through well-organized hard work. It is not surprising they feel that everyone should try harder to improve themselves. Says one of them, "I hate to see a gem in a poor setting. Imperfection calls to me. I can't avoid it."

Large intestine personalities enjoy participating in solid, well-grounded projects. In their full strength, they take life as it comes and follow through, no matter what it takes to get the best possible results. They know what must be eliminated, and what saved and nurtured for the best self to emerge. "At a lecture," says one of these discerning folk, " I will know quickly how the knowledge came to the speaker, and whether it has gone through inner processing. When I see flaws, I quietly take up the good and leave the rest, not judging the person or their work."

Even people of strong intestinal fortitude who are tired, whether young or old, will push harder than most to get a job done and try to find the perfect way to do so. A well-known children's story, "The Little Engine That Could," portrays a train that doubts it can climb a hill. On the slow track up the hill, it puffs, "I think I can, I think I can." Moving along, the determined little train gradually picks up speed. When anyone becomes sensitive to the tasks of the large intestine, they know what effort is required to get results. Very different from the rhythm of the small intestine, the pace of the large intestine tends toward slow but steady perseverance. These people love long-term projects with a steady momentum that, when completed, benefit others.

Disappointments fuel such people into action. They want to live beyond criticism, so as not to be negatively judged by anyone, especially themselves. As resistance arises, they make even more effort to follow through. They expect to work hard to attain the best possible results and become completely absorbed in the task at hand.

Those with healthy intestinal fortitude tend naturally to produce aesthetically superior results, no matter how much effort is required, because each detail of their handcraft or business is important to them. "I want to get it right and then I am satisfied," says an award-winning builder. "As a team we hold on until we get the results we set out to achieve." With a strong work ethic, these hardworking people appreciate the patient skillful workmanship of others. As they pursue excellence and inspire high standards, they are unusually conscientious in respecting the feelings of other people and sense when rewards are truly deserved. While performing specific tasks to their own best possible standard, they hold to their principles, like jewels, and keep employees involved in their ideals. Some invent exacting systems for exercise and precisely calibrated exercise machines. Others may build and set up their shops, studios, or offices with the finest materials they can find, regardless of cost. To fortify other people as well as themselves, they arrange their houses with jewel-like books and collections of statuary, stones, and textiles.

"Was I being specific enough?" they ask. With resolute patience for details, they are strong and steady housewives and parents, educators, musicians, architects, and real estate agents. Builders, plumbers, pipe-layers, and sanitation experts also exemplify intestinal fortitude. So do printers, craftspeople, and photo processors who relish bringing about good results. In full strength, the sublime power of manifestation hidden in the large intestine can build and maintain whole villages of substantial beauty with patient attentiveness to all the details involved.

Patient Genius with Details

M. C. Richards wrote a poem called "The Three Wisdoms":

"Go slow," said the snail.
"Hop hop," said the hare.
"Pace yourself," said the cheetah. "It's a long run."

Large intestine folk wait patiently and work late on their projects, after the large intestine fires in the afternoon, and tend to feel slower in the mornings. At ninety, my Aunt Edina still puts herself to work with patient determination every afternoon. Her workshop is filled with a large assortment of tools in drawers and moveable containers to assist her craftswoman's spirit with a never-ending throng of helter-skelter projects. She has gained a reputation for miles around for mending all sorts of broken things. Chairs and tables on their last legs become better than new. She collects glues and polishing waxes. One day as I watched her patiently put the perfect finishing touch on a cracked platter with dentist's glue, I realized how her whole workshop resembles the large intestine. I recognized the joy that glows through her as she transforms the discarded and dilapidated.

She says, "I like going to factories to see how things come about, how glass is cut, bread is packaged, and coffee is put in cans. I like to take battered tins and transform them into things of museum quality, even if it takes me years to do it. When I replace parts, I go to antique stores. I love slow transfiguration, bringing things to authentic beauty and finish."

A few years ago, as her backbone began to weaken and curve downward, she began to make lamps. Auctioneer for the mothers' club at a nearby school, she found a beautiful statuette, made a high bid, bashed down the gavel, and everyone was glad that it was hers. She took it home and cut wood for a simple lamp stand. Although she had never made a lamp before, she was never one to balk at an obstacle. She found tools and ran an electrical wire up though the lamp. Soon that first lamp was a whole piece, standing utterly upright, with a golden backbone to hold a bulb. She constructed her first lampshade to soften the bright glow that would wax and wane above the statue. Next, with hard-nosed pliers, she tightened a bright little finial above the place where the shade went down over the lamp head.

Then she heard herself saying, "I can make a better lamp than that." Several lamps later, Aunt Edina took an old-fashioned wrought-iron weighing scale with little movable weights to shift the balancing pans, cleaned the whole thing up, and oiled it with household oil. Then she measured, sawed, and sanded a sturdy platform, and inserted and bolted in a shining vertical lamp stand. She discovered automatic three-way "touch-tronic" switches. By putting one weight on the scale, the light turned on. Two weights brightened it. Three weights brought the pans into balance, and the lamp took on full luminescence! Now she felt the need to make a shade exactly to her liking. When this lamp was done, she made another like it for a couple who liked the first one. She never worked for money, yet now she was in business. She had a new reputation as a lamp maker.

My aunt's crumbling back continued to curve over. Battling on, she had operations to relieve the pain. Yet, day by day, in U formation, with the help of her canes, she walked with astonishing determination to her workshop. A neighbor helped her lift hugely weighty World War II bomb cartridges onto her worktable. Dark and tarnished, four feet tall, their forceful design had a certain beauty. She polished them up and varnished them until they shone like mirrors. She could see the war years reflected in them. She wired them inside and out with touch-tonic switches. She put bright white bulbs in them and stood back. By the time the black shades for those lamps were done, she had relived the wartimes of her life. To this day, those two lamps illuminate a dark wall in her living room, where they bring life and light.

And she keeps on, lamp by lamp. In the evenings, her work well done, she goes to her study to sit by the light of one of her creations. Guardian of the lamps, she curves deeply into a comfortable chair to brood a little and to knit.

FULFILLMENT THROUGH PRESERVING AND RESTORING

Marsha, a professional historical preservationist, also has a warm sense of achievement when work is well done. She loves the solid body of a railway station, a city plan, a house, as she strives to honor the "historical panorama" of individuals and craftsmanship that lives behind each. "I think of architectural environments as representative of the whole body and how well you treat yourself." She adds, "I am seldom satisfied because my attention is always going toward making things the best they can be."

When she is punching out walls or moving buildings to better locations, she dreads making "a really big mess." She struggles in the process to completion. "This too shall pass" are the four most important words in the English language, she says. "Worrying whether projects will come out perfectly is like constipation," she claims. She feels mounting creative power backing up within her as she works under time constraints, having a pressured feeling there is always much more work that could be done. The physical world moves too slowly for her. As she focuses on her goals, frustrations mount. "Details are a form of therapy, but when I work on one piece for too long and lose the overview because of too many details, I feel arthritic tension stymieing my joy in life." Yet, when all details fall into place at last, she feels waves of relief with her whole being.

PATTERNS OF REPETITION

Many such large-intestine stories are characterized by a growing sense of fullness and a corresponding apprehension as things build up, and then at last are released. A Ukrainian folktale reflects the large intestine's marvelous power of daily expansion, contraction, and releasing.

A young boy goes out to play in his brand-new fur-lined gloves. The sun is warm, so he puts them in his pocket. On his way home, he does not notice that one is missing.

Not long after, a mouse, looking for a warm place to spend the night, crawls inside the lost glove. It isn't long before a rabbit hops by. He wrinkles his nose and sees the mouse crouching inside. "Is there room for me too?" he cries.

"Oh, yes," says the mouse, "I'd be glad of company," and the rabbit snuggles in.

After a while an owl swoops down. "You two look very cozy in there. Is there a place for me too?"

"Of course," says the rabbit and the mouse. "Make yourself at home."

Some time later there comes a fox. "My, oh my," he says, "Why didn't you invite me to your party?"

"Well, c'mon in," they answer as one, "join us if you wish."

It is then that the badger turns up. "Humpf! Fun and games! No one told me about it. Typical. Well, I'll be on my way."

"No, no, no, Badger, we'll bunch up and fit you in. The glove has five fingers."

Then they hear heavy footsteps. It is Bear. "Fancy that, a glove. A perfect place to curl up and sleep for the winter."

"O Bear," cry the animals, "Take care. There are five of us in here."

"Plenty of room, plenty of room," says the bear, snuggling in.

And all would have been well if a passing flea had not decided to squeeze in too. It lands on bear's nose and crawls about, trying to find a place to settle down for the night. Bear tries to move his nose, but the flea goes on wriggling and Bear sneezes, "Ahhker-choo!" Out come the flea, the bear, the badger, the fox, the rabbit, and the mouse. And they all run home. The next morning the boy comes looking for his glove. He finds it all right, but what has happened to it only you and I know.

Versions of this tale exist in many languages to give children a reassuring sense of natural processes that they must engage in on a daily basis. Such stories, in combination with the observation of the comfortable rhythms of excretion experienced by animals, birds, and insects, have helped many children I know to accept themselves more fully.

A similar story tells of a man who lived with his wife and their children in a tiny house.

⊰⊱⊰⊱⊰⊱

Living Under Pressure

The family was always quarreling from the strain of living so closely together. One day the man could stand it no longer and went to a holy man to ask for advice.

"My dear fellow, do you have any chickens?" inquired the wise man.

"Yes," he replied.

"Excellent. Bring them into the house to live with you."

The discomfited man returned home and did as he was told. Now there were chickens underfoot and eggs in the bed. No one could sleep for the clucking sounds.

The desperate man returned to the holy one. "It was bad before," he exclaimed. "Now it is worse." "My friend, do you by any chance have a goat?"

"Yes," came the reply.

"Excellent. Then take the goat into the house to live with you."

Amazed at his advice, the man did as he was told. Now he was really in trouble. The goat went wild, butting everyone and everything. At last, the man returned. "Holy one, my life is in ruins. Please tell me what I must do."

"Do you by any chance have a cow," inquired the wise one.

"Yes," the man hesitantly replied.

"Then bring her in too."

Believing now that the old man must be mad, he obeyed nevertheless.

That night there was no room at all in the house. The cow could not even turn around. Feathers were in the soup, not to mention what was on the floor. The next day the man hardly dared return to his advisor, but he did.

Before he could speak, the wise man smiled with an infinitely patient look. "Go home now and take the animals out of your house."

The delighted man hurried back and did as he was told. That evening the whole family slept deeply. Returning, refreshed, the next day, he greeted the old master with joy. "How did you manage it? Last night nobody quarreled. We all slept well. There was so much room in our little house, it was a haven."

The holy one smiled and said, with a wink, "Remember, my friend, it could always be worse.

⁂

Getting Stuck in Details

A large-intestine personality often wants to put everything into perfect order under one roof, but cannot find enough room. As folk with intestinal fortitude hold high standards for complete success, they may pack collections of things into closets, bags, boxes, garages, attics, barns, whatever they can find to hold what might be useful to them. A woman in the process of spring-cleaning was purging drawers and closets. "Throw it away!" she said to her child, who asked, "Where's away?"

"I long for the Japanese approach to simplicity," said one of these large-intestine folk who had acquired substantial collections of many sorts. "I like comfortable, big, and spacious rooms with high ceilings and a view to the horizon, but I manage to fill them up quickly."

"I am a beachcomber, hunter, and gatherer," says another. "I just enjoy gathering and setting out beautiful things to have around me so I can feel their textures and colors viscerally." Says her good-natured husband, "Our life is like an antique shop where everything is crammed tightly together on floors, shelves, even up to the ceiling."

The collecting impulse can also manifest as clog and stubbornness. With the power to move mountains, these people tend to put things off, resist rush, and accumulate under high pressure a hopeless deadline feeling, brooding on the discomfort of these feelings as they mount up. "We often get bogged down," says a couple involved in many different projects and always having difficulty completing them. A calligrapher who illuminates sacred texts is often able to outwit her overwhelming expectations and her tendency to procrastinate. To protect herself from producing less than perfect results, she imagines a project already finished, and giving herself and others complete satisfaction.

The downside of the large-intestine pattern is obsessions and compulsions. A cautionary tale from India tells of the dangers of being unable to let go of projects and put them into a larger perspective.

⸙⸙⸙

The Potter's Wish

A potter aimed for perfection in all he did. One day as he prayed to Lord Shiva, there stood Lord Shiva himself in a brilliant beam of light. Shiva smiled and offered to fulfill the humble craftsman's greatest desire. The potter asked only that he would be able to make pots that would not chip, crack, or break.

Shiva granted this wish. The potter resumed his work and when he had finished the next pot, he dropped it to see if it would break. The pot remained whole. He threw it against a wall. No matter what he did, not even a scratch appeared on it.

Soon word spread about the potter's powers. People came from far and wide to buy his wares. His success gave him great happiness, until he learned that he was putting other potters out of business. Soon he, too, had very few customers.

Finally, the potter wept as he prayed. He asked himself, "How could I have created such a dilemma?"

Shiva again took pity on him and appeared again. The potter bowed low before him and said, "I see now that humans need imperfection in order to live. Please remove your gift." His wish was granted and, from that day on, the potter felt ecstatic gratitude at slight imperfections in his own work and in that of others.

⸙⸙⸙

The Healing Details of Family History

Achieving right relationship with one's family of origin and gaining historical perspective can be time-consuming and difficult, if not downright impossible. Nevertheless, large-intestine energies insist on the perfection that can only come through full understanding. Nora, a woman with abundant patience for details, wanted to get all of her relationships, including her relationship with the spiritual world, "right." Yet she was unable to share the past openly with many of the members of her large and troubled Italian family. After suffering a strange series of accidents around the time she turned fifty years old, her path led her to seek storytelling as a healing art.

She was puzzled and confused that her body had suddenly begun to stiffen and her spirit to grow hard and cold. As she was exploring her family history during a therapy session, she put together some of the details of her grandmother Bridget's story, and began consciously to feel her grandmother's unresolved rage within her own body and soul. One bright spring day when she appeared for a session, I told her I had dreamt the night before of her kneeling at an altar. This session was a turning point. Together we created a simple makeshift altar with a candle and a Bible. Nora lit the candle. Then to her astonishment, she opened the Bible exactly to her grandmother's favorite Psalm 91. She read it quietly.

"What shall I do now?" she asked.

"Why not tell your grandmother's story from beginning to end, from the time she was conceived until the time she died one hundred and one years later?" I suggested.

Nora protested that she did not know enough about her grandmother's story, although she was resolved to know more of the essential facts.

I said, "Just go ahead anyway."

So she began at the beginning, and many details that surprised her fell into place as she heard herself speak with new clarity and compassion about her grandmother's childhood. As she sought to see her grandmother's life as a whole, Nora realized for the first time with genuine astonishment that her grandmother had been born out of wedlock, and that was why her story had been suppressed.

This was a powerful realization, yet she calmly kept to her resolve. She realized clearly that, as a rejected orphan child in an Italian nunnery, Bridget had learned to sew to perfection. Nora spoke of Bridget's struggles in her new country, America, as she supported her ever-increasing family by sewing perfect garments for rich customers, while her husband philandered about town. She spoke of the bitterness that gathered in her grandmother's hands and heart until, when she was fifty, her arthritic fingers refused to sew one stitch more. Crippled, she sat for fifty-one more years, holding court over the whole family with tenacious rage.

As Nora spoke about her hardworking, perfectionistic grandmother, great pity and tenderness filled her heart. The story unfolded steadily until the day of her grandmother's death and funeral. More hidden details came to light and fell into place. Then Nora read her grandmother's favorite Psalm 91 again and closed the Bible. A great blessing filled the air. The new peace that surrounded her seemed palpable. Understanding awakened as she felt more compassion for her own relentless and raging drive to perfection.

On her way home after the session during which these events unfolded, Nora realized it was her grandmother's birthday. She resolved to set up an altar at home in her own workspace to remember the more complete details of her grandmother's story with an understanding heart. She carried the details with care and newfound maturity when, a few months later, she took her daughter with her to Italy to visit the sites of her grandmother's childhood. She was drawn to experiences that helped her further release the burden she had carried for so many years, and she, her daughter, and other family members began to live with new freedom.

GIVING BACK FULLY

A story from India portrays the desire to give earthly accomplishments back full circle to their spiritual origin:

❧❧❧

The Image Maker

A sculptor was famous throughout the land for his perfectly beautiful bronze statues of Shiva. The spirit of Shiva lived in every one of them. The sculptor refused to sell the statues, but instead gave them away to the temples, to journeying monks, and to ordinary people who needed them. In return, his village kept him alive with lentils and vegetables, and gave him a comfortable little room to live and work in. He was one of those rare people who could be considered completely happy.

One day, the king and his procession were passing through the village to give the people a view of the royal grandeur and to brighten their dull lives. The king saw the Shiva images and was amazed.

The next day the king sent a messenger to buy a statue. The messenger held out a bag of gold. But the sculptor was unaccustomed to the offer of gold. The messenger said he could not refuse the king's money, threw it at him, and sped away with the statue.

The artist tried to return to work and put the incident behind him. But from that day, to his horror, every statue he made looked like the king. In dismay, he melted them down and tried again, but the same thing happened.

Finally, he went to the village guru and told him his problem. "I am deeply offended by the king!" the artist exploded.

"Ahhh!" said the teacher, "When your resentment is stronger than your love, you create what you hate."

After some meditation, the image maker knew what he had to do. He took his clothes, his begging bowl, and the bag of gold. Day after day he walked, begging in the rain, sleeping in temples, and guarding the bag of gold, until he arrived at the capital.

When he knocked on the palace door and asked to see the king, the guards laughed and told him that the king did not receive beggars. But after days and weeks, the king finally noticed this persistent mendicant and agreed to speak with him.

"Your majesty, I am a humble image maker. Some time ago you sent a messenger to me to buy an image. I am honored, your majesty, but I cannot sell them. Those images come to me as a gift from Shiva."

And he held out the bag of gold.

The king, seeing the expression on the image maker's face, took the gold back. Then he sent the image maker home by royal caravan.

The image maker returned to his hut. People asked him about his journey, but he could not wait to get back to work. He carved a fresh image, created the mold, poured and let the metal cool, and then set to work polishing the bronze. It began to glow like the sun. To his relief, he once more held in his hands the serene countenance of Shiva.

❧❧❧

Transformational Storytelling

Large Intestine Affirmation

Life perfects itself through me.

Basic Large Intestine Story Dynamic

Resistance turns into radiant accomplishments.

Large Intestine Protagonists and Antagonists

Large intestine protagonists (characters who support large intestine health) are conscientious and self-disciplined, with strong convictions. They strive to be objective, thorough, and cheerful. With intuitive belly knowledge, they recognize how situations can be improved. With an overriding sense of responsibility, guided by a higher purpose, they tend to be humane, generous, and realistic.

Large intestine antagonists (characters who express large intestine dysfunction) are obsessive about imperfections and wrongs, dissatisfied, scolding, workaholic, overly fastidious, and critical of themselves and others. Impeding life, they become dreamy, sluggish, and pressured as they accumulate and hold on to more and more possessions, beyond what they need or can use.

Basic Story Elements

Myths and stories often resonate with specific internal processes. This reliable pattern invokes well-being and resilience in every cell of your body:

Setting Out: The protagonist sets out in quest of greater love, strength, justice, wisdom, and happiness.

Trouble: One or more obstacles and/or antagonists interfere with the journey.

Help: Wise and benevolent help comes, often giving a gift.

Positive Ending: The protagonist fulfils the quest with joy and celebration.

SUMMONING YOUR STORYTELLER

Storytellers with intestinal fortitude take a strong stand. In their desire for a perfect ending, they tend to be acutely aware of details, as they slowly and thoroughly push through to a strong and soul-satisfying denouement. Breathing and speaking from the belly, they elaborate with dream-like ease as they assemble a jeweled tapestry of characters and events. Their stories may take a long time to recount, with many pauses, as they seek that moment of a perfect ending. They may use pointer finger or place thumb and pointer together as they give precise attention to each detail and word.

Exercises to Explore and Balance the Large Intestine

Transforming compulsions and obsessions. Imagine in detail an antagonist who embodies one or more of the traits listed. Turn yourself into this character as you walk about the room. Now write or tell a story in which your antagonist meets a protagonist who embodies one or more of the virtues listed. In your story, let the protagonist prevail. Celebrate your story by sharing it with at least one other person. Or imagine a very satisfying ending for a tale that has not yet been told.

Seeking perfection. The Sufi poet Hafiz wrote: "What power is it in our sinew and mind / that will not die / that keeps us shopping for the perfect dress?" Tell about your adventures looking for the perfect shoes or garments to wear on a special occasion. Look at anything in your immediate surroundings, point at it, and consider as many ways as you can to improve it.

Going beyond "I can't." Characters who hesitate and hold back are often found in stories. Think of a habit you would like to transform in a way that would give you great satisfaction. Tell the story of someone who first says, "I can't," but through the process of doing, succeeds like "The Little Engine That Could." Let strong willpower bring your character through the adventure.

Tell about a time when you found such an engine of power within you.

Accumulation for the fun of it. Many people enjoy collecting jewelry, pottery, antique furniture, old clothes and shoes, and other memorabilia. Design a museum or other architectural space to hold a variety of fine items of which you or someone else is fond.

For comic relief from obsessions and perfectionism, try telling a never-ending story with friends, such as "I packed my grandmother's bag and in it I put…" Just keep adding a little more to the original story each time, gradually accumulating more and more details to remember and to keep in order. Be sure to unpack the whole bag in reverse order before the game ends.

Imagine you are going on a long journey and discover at the airport that you are allowed only one piece of luggage, instead of the two you brought. How would you manage this situation?

Imagine a girdle of power. Design and draw in detail a belt of power to wear at the level of the transverse colon, just above the belly button. Imagine yourself wearing this belt as you work, or giving it away as an empowering gift to someone else. Of what metal is it forged? What jewels and gemstones are fastened to it? Show off your girdle by rising up and describing it and the inspired workmanship that manifested it. Soul qualities resonate with gems and metals, whether gold or steel, onyx or opal. What powers are communicated to both body and soul through these substances? Give gratitude to each one, and through the power of your imagination return each respectfully to the earth.

Completing and renewing. Think of an unsatisfying situation in your life. Imagine throwing it into a compost heap, where it will gradually turn into a great treasure. Visualize that treasure and the healthy satisfaction it will give in time.

Expanding Large Intestine Awareness Through Dance, Music, and Yoga

Dance

In a seated dance, twist one leg around the other and secure it with your toes pressed against the calf of the stationary leg. Cross the opposite elbow over the arm that is the same as your crossing leg, and press your palms together. Hold these twists as you sway and bend. Then rise, relax, and freely express this digestive power, especially attending to your shoulders, lower torso, and legs. Visualize each movement with the intention of expressing it warmly, fully, and perfectly.

Suggested music

Brahms, *Fifty-One Exercises, Waltz no. 11*
Fauré, Pavane, op. 50

Yoga asanas (Sanskrit names in italics)

Lateral Angle *(Parsvakonasana)*
Warrior 2 and Reverse Warrior *(Virabhadrasana)*
Wind Removing *(Pavanamuktasana)*
Eagle *(Garuasana)*
Wide-Legged Goddess Squat *(Malasana)*

6

Inspiring Leader: The Lungs

A young schoolteacher dreamed that an angel appeared to her saying, "You will be given a child who will grow up to become a world leader." The teacher awoke in a cold sweat and with a new sense of responsibility. She took a large breath and gradually began to formulate a plan. From that day forward, her teaching changed. Each young person who walked through her classroom became for her a potential world leader, and she taught as if the future of the world depended on her lessons.

It is not surprising that expanded breaths can profoundly change our relationship with reality. The lung meridian ranges widely within the torso. Originating just under the diaphragm, it plunges into the region of the large intestine, and then rises toward the lungs and throat, to branch out toward sensitive points just beneath the clavicle. Then it flows down the inner arms into the thumbs, emerging at the inside of each thumbnail.

Firmly trace the path of your lung meridian. To inspire the resolve of a fully motivated teacher, go for a brisk early morning walk, or jog in place for a while. Inhale magnificently and hold this in-breath for a few moments as you feel your chest muscles and shoulders relax and expand. Imagine living for a whole lifetime with such an exhilarating chest expansion each time you take a breath. To stimulate more inbreathing, do an ordinary push-up. Or do a standing push-up by stepping into a open doorway, the top of which is not too high for you to reach. Press upward against the top support of the doorway, while at the same time pushing down strongly against the floor. Or do push-ups against a wall. When I discovered how deflated my lungs often are during

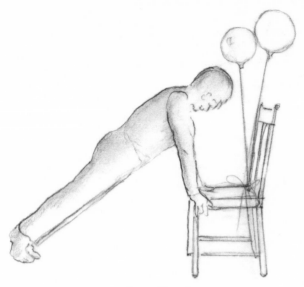

Lung Exercise

the workday, I rejoiced to discover the effects of these simple exercises.

As the lungs move in relationship with all that breathes, physical forces that can deeply affect our thoughts and resolves quicken throughout the body. Every minute, the short rhythmic pulsations of our breathing produce, on average, eight rounds of inhalations and exhalations that dissolve into the surrounding atmosphere. Deep complete breathing can produce the glorious feeling of being in touch with and empowered by breathing far greater than our own. Sublimely fertile breaths live in the mysteries of time and space. The ancient Indians sang of Brahma, the Creator, breathing forth the entire universe, the world story. Is it any wonder that those who live especially in the sway of the lungs often feel an expansive, even intoxicating, and colossal sense of purpose?

With upbeat emotions and a sense of global reach and grip, lung-strong people devise initiatives of magnitude and momentum and inspire others to cooperate. When informed and guided by moral principles in a culture of generosity and love, their projects greatly benefit humankind. Yet they can also bring about catastrophes of monumental proportions.

Lung-predominant people are exuberant, physically robust city planners, real estate agents, or politicians, who with pomp and ceremony inspire empire-building. Strong leaders also often work backstage to support large and ambitious projects. A day is immense for them. They may gladly work two or three jobs as, like the Greek hero Jason, they move through, over, under, and around all obstacles in their quest for whatever "golden fleece" is their goal. They may organize large projects and conferences in their spare time. They can be warmly persuasive salespeople, who tend to get what they want and lead us to spend too much.

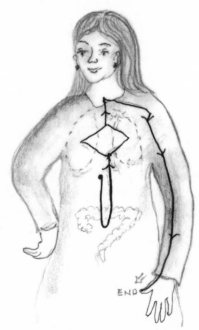

The Lung Meridian

To be supported by the healthy lung personality is like having an infusion of oxygen. A friend of mine who exemplifies the lung personality is a natural leader. Quests of mythic dimensions stir in the wellspring of her soul. With a strong constitution and the support of oxygen, as a community leader, she takes in others' needs and viewpoints. Then with expansive generosity, she acts to help them overcome their sorrows, generating funding and all the necessary leadership and support for projects to succeed. "We'll raise the money!" is her motto. She has built a park in her neighborhood and a home for battered children, and given sturdy inspirational hope to local politics. She is undaunted by expenses, real estate needs, or the challenge of caring for her large family, house, and garden.

Along with powers of leadership, the lungs also support prowess of memory and musicality. As chest and sinuses circulate fresh air through the body, awesome physical power rises to support speaking and singing. Our lungs are moist, malleable, and finely coordinated with the larynx, the most rapidly moving and flexible muscle in the body. Breathing instigates the sheer stamina required in the world's performing arenas. A strong stomach supports the lungs in a reciprocal action to create a powerful need to vocalize. As upper and lower bodies listen to each other, balancing many rhythms of both body and soul, music sounds forth. Inspired by lung circulation, whether Balkan, Brazilian, or Szechuan, the intensity of the human voice requires the participation of the whole orchestra of the body. Strong vocalists and speakers the world over lift strength from the earth up through their lungs and throats into the resonating sinus chambers in their heads. As they breathe deeply and harmoniously, their voices, like yours, can release rapture. Try speaking the following tale aloud.

❧❀❧❀❧

The Girl Who Loved the North Wind

Once there was a girl whose lover was the North Wind. He lived far away but once a year came to visit her. All year she waited for him. She waited for him in the woods. She waited for him on the hills. She watched for him on the surface of the river far below, for that was the path he took. Yes, every year he came whirling up the river and stopped off to make love to the wild girl of the woods, and all year she waited for him.

But one year he did not come, and the girl waited and worried. Did he have another girlfriend? She asked the warm South Wind if he knew. She asked the West Wind and the East Wind, but they all were silent.

So the girl went to her grandmother. The old lady listened as only a wise old woman can, and she offered to teach her a song. "I know a song," she said, "so powerful that when he hears it, he will have to come. After you have learned it, go to the top of the hill and sing."

When the girl learned the song, she climbed to the top of the hill, high above the forest. With her eyes on the river, she started singing, and when she finished her song she waited, but nothing happened. Not a leaf stirred, not a bird sang. So she sang again, but again nothing happened. Her singing was sad, and hot air and dust caked her throat.

She returned to her grandmother and told her that the song magic did not work. The North Wind had not come.

The old woman looked her up and down, as only a wise old woman can, and said, "Little wonder he did not come. Look at yourself. Your clothes, your hair, your face. Go bathe in the river, comb out your hair, and when you sing, throw back your head. Sing loud—sing as if you are expecting him."

So the girl went down to the river and washed herself. She scraped her body clean with stones and rubbed it with oil. She combed out her long hair until it glistened. Then she put on her old clothes, climbed up the hillside, and started to sing. But her song was still not strong enough and nothing happened. Then she noticed the old clothes she was still wearing. "He will never come to me if I am dressed like this," she said, as she stepped out of those tattered garments. Now she stood before the world, naked and beautiful. And then she threw back her head. This time her voice rang out strong and rich and clear as she sang, until every part of her being glowed with joy.

Suddenly, the face of the river trembled. The trees on its banks began to sway. The branches shook and the leaves quivered, for the North Wind was coming. Round the bend of the river he came. Down from the sky he came. Swooping up the hillside, he came racing. He took the girl in his arms and wrapped himself about her. She took him down into the woods, and there they made love. When he was gone, the girl lay for a long time on the hills, softly singing the song that had called him to her. And every year after that, she prepared herself as the old woman had told her to do. She washed herself in the river, stepped out of her old clothes, and threw back her head to sing, to sing loud.

<hr/>

The Breath of Children

Whether we are young or old, as we harness this power and our breathing joins with our heart's desires and morality, great inner strength can be achieved. A socially conscious couple in their eighties has learned to sit regularly and do a breathing meditation. As they inhale, they say, "I am at peace," and as they exhale, "I am strong." As babies we learn to scream with joy, and also at any threat to life. Breath and speech help us to make demands and commands. Muscular impulses that coordinate with our breath metabolize air within the whole body, and eventually help us form words and notes. Adding breath to the soul and spirit enables us to think magnificent and sometimes transcendent thoughts that are supported by the strength of the whole body.

For both children and the adults who care for them, stories can provide a calming environment, as full and steady breathing does during meditation. A kindergarten teacher who wanted to strengthen and balance the lungs of the children in her care made up a tale for her class about an old couple who every autumn gathered twigs and twine and made a cage. Then they called wild birds into the cage and carefully took care of them in the warmth of their home. As the green buds of spring began to open, they released the birds back to the wild forest. The whole class found much pleasure in acting out this little tale many times.

Inspired by the benefits from this story, the teacher decided to create a story for a troubling boy in her class. He was big and strong but he was also clumsy in his movements and careless of others. His mother tended to be permissive because she feared her son's anger, which reminded her of her own traumatic childhood. The teacher's story helped the boy, his mother, and the whole classroom of children to change.

The Boy Who Lived with Giants

Once a baby boy was born into a loving family. During one of their journeys, the baby was lost. Some giants found the human child and took care of him. He grew strong and healthy. One day the giants saw some humans traveling across their land and thought that the boy should be returned to his own people.

The people gladly took the boy with them, but when they arrived at their village, they quickly saw by his behavior that the boy was used to living with giants and had learned to move in their clumsy way. He often bumped into things and pushed people out of his way without showing any respect for their feelings. The children of the village complained of his rough ways. When mothers saw him coming, they avoided him, hurrying away with their children. The boy's heart became so sad and lonely that one day he wandered into the forest near his home, sat on a rock, and began to cry.

Suddenly, there appeared a beautiful old woman who put her hand on his shoulder. "Don't worry," she said, "you can come to live with us. We will teach you our ways."

So he lived with the wise woman and her people. And when he was ready, he returned to his village, where everyone was surprised to see how graceful and patient he had become. Soon he was dearly loved by all and cherished for his generosity.

Imagination can connect growing children with streaming healing support. A child who was born of several generations of coal miners and who had suffered from severe asthma from the time he was born went through many changes when his mother decided to become his personal storyteller. Exhausted from the suggestions of many zealous friends who wanted to help, this mother, with a little encouragement, began trusting her own intuition. One early spring morning, after a succession of sleepless nights, when she was on the verge again of driving their son to the hospital, her husband suggested, "Maybe it's time for a story." The tired mother looked at her husband, and took a deep breath. This was the beginning of a new way of life, even during the boy's full-blown asthma attacks. As the first of her stories ended, her son's breathing had changed and he was able to go to sleep. Creatures with strong breath became helpful story entities for this family. The mother believes that her son survived his earlier years through the stories they wove together, and the paintings and drawings he made at all hours of the day and night to discharge, contain, and embody them.

FINDING AND CLAIMING POWER

A flowing sense of wholeness arises through storytelling that supports health of body and soul in people of any age. All our organs are instruments of our souls. A professional artist dreaded the years ahead with her budding adolescent children. She joined a healing story group because she wanted to free her imagination to help her to cope. She was astonished to find herself writing a story about royalty on a high mission:

> The king and his men astride their strong horses, bodies bent to the wind, traversed an arid inhospitable plain for many months with little food or water. The king spurred them on, reminding himself and them of their great mission and the good citizens who relied on them. Each one of them was brave, battling this hostile land. Some succumbed to death from snakebites and starvation or illness. Still, the king pushed onward. At last he saw the magnificent mountain range that he had been seeking, with its grand vista. He drew his men toward it. Inspired, they rode, their banners and hair blowing in the wind, counting the miles by the rhythmic galloping of their horses' great hooves.

The mother reported that after these images came to her and she wrote them down, she felt uplifted and stronger. She remembered more clearly the challenges of her own adolescence and took a long and more hopeful view of the new terrain she and her husband had before them.

As each inhalation and exhalation impacts countless other rhythms wound into the clockwork of our bodies, lung strength arouses a natural drive for leadership and power. Healthy lungs and a balanced mind generate wisely interdependent leadership. Canada geese tell a continuous story of shared leadership as they migrate over long distances. When the lead goose gets tired, it rotates back into the formation, and another goose flies to the point position in the V formation. It is sensible to take turns sharing the hard and demanding tasks. When a goose flies out of formation, it suddenly feels the resistance of trying to go it alone. It quickly gets back into formation to take advantage of the buoying power of the bird in front of it. As each bird flaps its wings, it creates an uplift for the bird immediately following. By flying in V formation, the whole flock has greater flying range than if each bird flew on its own. Geese honk from behind to encourage those up front to keep up their speed. When one gets sick, wounded, or shot down, two other geese will drop out of formation and follow it down to lend help and protection. They stay with the fallen goose until it is able to fly again or dies. Then they launch out on their own, or with another V formation, to catch up with their flock.

Belinda says to Dorothy in *The Wizard of Oz*, "You've always had the power!" Yet whenever we feel that other people are stealing our air to increase their own, our personal and collective life stories deflate. Awareness is dulled, memory unreliable. We are fortunate to find a way to put our feet down, find our voices again, and the spirit of hope and joy within us. A Tamil story from India tells of a poor widow who discovered unexpected power hidden in her breath and words as she spoke her truth.

⚜⚜⚜⚜⚜

The Story Behind the Sorrow

Once a widow lived with her grown children and their families. All of them scolded and ill-treated her. As her spirit shrank, her body grew fatter to soften the blows of their behavior. She had no one to whom she could turn and share her troubles. One day in her sorrow, she left the house and wandered until at last she found herself inside a small, crumbling, roofless house. Through her tears, she found herself speaking her grievances to one of its cracked walls. Suddenly, the wall collapsed and crashed to the ground at her feet. Gradually, she noticed that her body felt lighter, so she turned to another wall and spoke more of her grievances. As she found words for more of the abuse she had endured, down came that wall, and she felt lighter still. Now she turned to the third wall with the truth of the cruelties that had been inflicted on her, which she had carried silently for so long. Down came the third wall also and turned to rubble. One wall remained. When she turned toward the fourth wall, she could hear the outrage in her voice as she spoke. As that wall collapsed too, she felt stronger than she had ever felt before. There she stood in the crumpled old house, astonished, triumphant, released from her burdens, the rubble of so many sad years at her feet. And with newfound determination, she walked out of that place briskly, with her head held high.

⚜⚜⚜⚜⚜

When the widow spoke her backed-up sorrows, she expressed the hidden mettle of her inner self. This sent messages to her whole body. As she remembered herself, she gathered dignity. By expressing respect for herself, she was on the path that disarms and transforms bullies.

DEALING WITH TYRANTS: TIPS FROM STORIES

Virtues and hazards connected with the powers of the lungs are expressed in myths, fairy tales, and in everyday news stories throughout the world. Moving from contraction to exhilaration, inflated breath can lead to antics that "blow away" others with good-humored laughter. Relating "tall tales" and "fish stories" can be an amusing pastime. The delight of exaggerated words riding on big breaths has inspired annual public competitions in many lands that draw huge crowds in many lands. During these events, storytellers sometimes stand before a panel of judges and devise fantastical tales delivered with lung-strong bombast and bluster. Yet as forceful words disconnect more and more from truth, the quest for power and success can, in reality, backfire in terrible deeds. Natural leaders can achieve positive results, yet also flatten and even brutally destroy without a qualm what does not conform to their will. Impressive manipulations and belligerent disrespect for others, in public and in private life, call continuously for another kind of story that holds all life to be sacred.

When the energy of the lungs has not circulated through the heart's wisdom, it often has a treacherous effect. Many personalities in whom lungs prevail for better and for worse are infamous in the annals of war. As their chests and egos swell, their capacity for heartfelt thought dims. Windbags and bulldozers, they can bully others into breathless submission, the way a dirigible casts an eerie shadow over a landscape. They intimidate others to prevent them from speaking back and asking questions such as: What are you doing? Why did you say that? How can I help you see the effect of your words and deeds?

Stories and storytellers naturally arise to counter abusive domination and harmonize the bodily functions that support and restore healthier perspectives. A Br'er Rabbit story from the African American tradition reflects the highest expression of the lungs, and also its downside. Brother Rabbit champions his people in the story with witty good humor. A good leader who is playfully in touch with his heart, he skillfully shows others how to stand up successfully to a self-serving bully.

⁕⁕⁕⁕⁕

Br'er Rabbit and Br'er Tiger

During a famine, a great big Bengal Tiger claimed the only running water and the only fruit-bearing tree in the territory. When the creatures came looking for nourishment, this tyrant rose and said, "Wumpf! Wumpf! I'll eat you up if you come here."

All the creatures were too scared to say anything to Br'er Tiger. They backed off, crawled to the edge of the woods, and sat there with misery in their eyes. They were so starved and so parched that their ribs showed through their hides and their tongues hung out of their mouths.

But then Br'er Rabbit came along. After sizing up the situation, the friendly rabbit jumped on a stump so that all could see him. They crowded round as he whispered his plan to them. Next morning, just before daybreak, all the big and little creatures gathered and took their posts.

Then Br'er Rabbit came down the road with a long grass rope wrapped round his shoulder, singing: "Oh Lord, oh Lord, there's a great big wind that's a coming through the woods, and it's going to blow all the people off the Earth!"

That was the signal for all the animals to make a huge racket that sounded like a cyclone was coming through the woods, flapping their wings and shaking the big trees and the bushes while Br'er Bear beat on a hollow log. Then all the animals started hollering: "Br'er Rabbit, I want you to tie me. I don't want that big wind to blow me off the Earth!"

The great big Bengal Tiger begged Br'er Rabbit to tie him down too, but Br'er Rabbit coolly replied, "I don't have time to tie you, Br'er Tiger. I've got to go down the road to tie up those other folks to keep the wind from blowing them off the Earth."

When the terrified Tiger started begging, Br'er Rabbit repeated: "I don't have time to bother with you. I have to go tie those other folks, I told you."

"I don't care about those other folks," said Br'er Tiger. "I want you to tie me so the wind won't blow *me* off the Earth."

The windy racket kept getting louder and louder and pretty soon Br'er Rabbit had his grass rope tied around the tiger's neck and feet, and the Tiger was calling for him to tie him tighter. So Br'er Rabbit wrapped him around and around so tight that Br'er Tiger couldn't move. Then Br'er Rabbit called to all the creatures to come and look. "Hush your fuss, children. Stop all your crying. Come over here and look. There's our great big tiger. He had all the juicy fruit and all the drinking water, enough for everybody. But he wouldn't give a bite of food or a drop of water to anybody, no matter how much they needed it."

After the animals had filled their sacks and buckets, they all joined in a song of thanks for their leader, Br'er Rabbit, who had helped them work together to tie the tiger.

⊶⊷⊶⊷⊶⊷

Sacred Transformations

Although healthy lung personalities are naturally attracted to the most powerful positions, they can also empower others to become more powerful. They often serve the strongest people until they themselves attain their full strength. The legend of Saint Christopher exemplifies their strength of will and growing consciousness. His story is included in The Golden Legend, a medieval collection of saints' legends.

⊶⊷⊶⊷⊶⊷

The Legend of Saint Christopher

Reprobus was a Canaanite of huge stature, fearful face, and rough ways. He longed to serve and obey the most powerful master in the world. Seeing his king make the sign of the cross whenever the name of the devil was uttered, he deemed the devil more mighty than the king, and went to serve the devil. After a time, he saw the devil fleeing from a stone cross in the desert. He inquired about the meaning of the cross, and then he knew Christ to be more powerful than any devil, and so he went to seek Him.

After much wandering, he met a hermit. "Stay awake, pray, and serve," said the hermit, who then directed him to a river where many had perished. Said the hermit, "I hope He shall show Himself to thee."

Reprobus went to the river and made a dwelling for himself. With the help of a huge pole for balance, he carried all manner of people safely across the rushing waters. After many years of faithful service to travelers, one night as the ferryman lay sleeping, he heard the voice of a child calling, "Bring me over."

He awoke, but at first he could see no one who needed transport over the river. Only on the third call did he at last discover a child who was standing at the edge of the rushing water. He willingly lifted the child onto his shoulders, took up his staff, and entered the river to cross it. As the water rose, the child seemed to grow heavier and heavier. The faithful ferryman feared they both would drown. He groaned, "Child, thou weighest almost as though I had all the world upon me." In the swirling, surging currents, sometimes carrying the child above his head in his upstretched hands, the ferryman just managed to reach the other shore. At last, at the far side of the river, the child revealed his true identity.

"I am He on whom rests all the sorrows of humankind," He said. "Return home and set thy staff in the earth by thy house. Tomorrow thou shalt see that it lives."

When the ferryman awoke the next day, his staff had become a living tree laden with leaves and fruit. Then the hermit gave him a new name appropriate to his bearing. Christophorus means "he who bears the Christ." He soon set out to teach the world, carrying the Christ Child with him in his soul, bringing much sorrow to light, and blessing many to new spiritual awareness through his prayers and good works.

⁕⁘⁕⁘⁕

A sacred teaching tale from China also exemplifies the ambition and capacity for utmost spiritual power that is stored in our lungs and breathing when they are joined with devotion and do not shirk the immeasurable grief caused by human behavior. The legend of Kwan Yin contains both negative and positive lung energy. The king's daughter received her spiritual name when she had attained her ultimate goal: the power to alleviate every sort of suffering.

The Legend of Kwan Yin

A notorious king killed thousands in war for his own satisfaction and went on ruling with his queen for many years. They longed in vain for an heir. At last the king resorted to prayer, requesting that both Buddhist and Taoist priests pray for seven days and seven nights in order that they should obtain a son. When the period was over, the king and queen went in person to the temple to offer sacrifices to the god of the sacred mountain of their kingdom.

The mountain god did not altogether reject their prayers. He ordered messengers to seek a worthy person who was on the point of being reincarnated back into the earthly world. In a small village, the royal messengers found a good man whose ancestors had observed all the ascetic rules of the Buddhist faith for three generations. This man was the father of three sons. Long before, he had refused to shelter a famous robber and his men, and his entire household had been burned with everyone and everything in it. Now the three sons of this good man were permitted to be born again to the royal couple as three daughters.

The king named the third daughter Miao Shan. From the time she was born, she manifested great virtue. She told her sisters that she desired nothing more than to reach such a high degree of goodness that she might travel throughout the universe to save the spirits that do evil, and cause them to do good. She said, "That is my only ambition."

Eventually, the king and queen sought husbands for their three daughters. They wanted to find a man capable of ruling the kingdom as the king's successor.

"I do not wish to marry," said Miao Shan. "I wish to attain Buddhahood, and I promise I will not be ungrateful to you."

Like Shakespeare's King Lear, mad with rage, her father shouted, "Wicked imbecile! How dare you contradict my will?"

But Miao Shan quietly replied, "My wish is to heal humanity of all its ills through kindness."

With that, the king commanded his palace guards to take away her court robes and to drive her away. Miao Shan quickly asked her father's permission to retire to a nunnery in a neighboring province in which a multitude of nuns lived together in prayer. The king commanded these good women to give his royal daughter the most difficult and demaning tasks. Miao Shan faithfully strove to fulfill each one. Because she was so willing, the Master of Heaven sent heavenly spirits to help her perform her duties, so that she could give herself to the pursuit of perfection without neglecting her practical tasks.

When the mother superior of the nunnery sent word to the king that his daughter was receiving celestial help, the king was furious. He ordered infantry and cavalry to surround the nunnery and to burn it to the ground, with the nuns inside. The others nuns complained bitterly to Miao Shan, saying, "It is you who have brought upon us this terrible disaster." The doomed nuns invoked the aid of heaven and earth, and soon their profound prayers caused a storm to quench the fire. Hearing of this miracle, the king ordered his daughter to be brought to him in chains, to be executed. But, again through divine intervention, the sword of the executioner broke in two and other weapons turned against Miao Shan also fell to pieces.

Suddenly, a heavenly tiger leapt into the scene of execution, dispersed the executioners, took the inanimate body of Maio Shan on his back, and disappeared into the deep forest lands beyond. There her soul was met by a celestial being dressed in blue, shining with brilliant light, and carrying a large banner. Together in a troupe they traveled through the infernal regions, where the condemned souls were released from chains to listen to her prayers. No sooner had she finished praying than hell transformed into a paradise of joy. The instruments of torture there were transformed into flowers.

Then the soul of the princess was returned with great celebration to the forest land to reenter her body. At last the Buddha appeared to her and invited her to an ancient monastery on an island. This island was inhabited only by Immortals. After nine years in that holy place, Miao Shan attained her ultimate goal, and was enthroned, so that the whole world might benefit from her spiritual attainment. The Dragon-king of the Western Sea, the gods of the Five Sacred Mountains, the emperor-saints, the officials of the Ministry of Time, the Celestial Functionaries in charge of wind, rain, thunder, and lightning—all these and many more arrived as Miao Shan took her seat on the lotus throne. The Immortals assembled there then proclaimed her sovereign of Heaven and Earth, and a Buddha. She received her new name, Kwan Yin, which she bears to this day.

Afterward, by her power of devotion and willing sacrifice, she completely transformed her tyrannical father, at last, into a man of compassion, and her mother the queen also became wise.

༺ⵢ༄ⵢ༄ⵢ༄༻

Transformational Storytelling
Lung Affirmation
I breathe the power of peace.

Basic Lung Story Dynamic
Egocentric ambition becomes enlightened leadership.

Lung Protagonists and Antagonists

Lung protagonists (characters who support lung health) defend the oppressed. They are exhilarating leaders, who rise up again and again like a phoenix. They are sturdy, zealous, and forceful, with strong will and memory, and tend to work on a grand scale.

Lung antagonists (characters who express lung dysfunction) are explosively hostile, hard-hearted, argumentative, and bossy. Avoiding their own sorrows, they can become malicious bullies given to blind rage, megalomania, and lies.

Basic Story Elements

Myths and stories often resonate with specific internal processes. This reliable pattern invokes well-being and resilience in every cell of your body:

Setting Out: The protagonist sets out in quest of greater love, strength, justice, wisdom, and happiness.

Trouble: One or more obstacles and/or antagonists interfere with the journey.

Help: Wise and benevolent help comes, often giving a gift.

Positive Ending: The protagonist fulfils the quest with joy and celebration.

SUMMONING YOUR STORYTELLER

Storytellers with predominant lung energy empower others. As they speak, weaknesses evaporate. Their voices vibrate with strong will and have a rousing effect, like the trumpets, horns, and trombones in the brass section in an orchestra, which require strong breath. Lung-strong people know how to use words and pauses to bring about more effective action from their listeners. They inspire others with their anecdotes and stories. These storytellers tend to dress with padded shoulders, strong shoes, and empowering colors and style. Their physical presence is unapologetic. Their characteristic gestures are definite and commanding.

Exercises to Explore and Balance the Lungs

Greet your lungs. Look in a mirror and wave a grand hello to yourself. Straighten your shoulders strongly and squarely, flare your nostrils, and breathe in slowly through your nose. Hold the inhalation and give yourself time to commune with this clear and powerful breath until you feel ready to converse with your lungs. Find out how they feel about the life you are leading now. A woman who was constantly working to support worthy projects spoke to her lungs and was surprised when they said, "Have a rest!"

Empowering breaths. To discover more of this storyteller within you, inhale a long, strong breath. Go outside and sing to the earth and skies. Listen to what comes back to you, and rises from deep within you. Fill yourself with a feeling of overriding power. Look out on everything as if it is part of your growing realm of influence. See yourself surrounded by a strong, capable, well-trained team that you command. Place your heels, your lower legs, your palms, and the back of your head against a wall. With your eyes closed, lean back and allow an entire wall to support you. All this behind you is your territory, your country, your birthright. Imagine it is ten yards, two miles, fifty miles. Walk forward, looking actively ahead, carrying the sense of command. Then recite this nursery rhyme a few times:

> The grand old duke of York
> He had 10,000 men.
> He marched them up to the top of the hill,
> And marched them down again.
>
> And when they were up, they were up.
> And when they were down, they were down.
> And when they were only halfway up
> They were neither up nor down.

Create characters to balance the lungs. To engage the dynamic energies of your lungs, breathe in fully, hold your breath for a few seconds, and allow your imagination to show you a character that embodies this inflated condition. Now breathe out and pause for a few moments before inhaling. What kind of deflated characters appear to your imagination?

Make up a brief "Once upon a time" story in which a protagonist and an antagonist embodying some of the characteristics summarized meet. By the end of your story, let the protagonist prevail.

Describe lung-dominant characters in your life. A healthy lung personality honors the boundaries of others and empowers them to worthy leadership. Describe someone you know who is committed to a noble cause and is trusted as a good leader. A supreme example of this is the figure of Aslan the lion in *The Chronicles of Narnia*. Then describe an unbalanced lung personality—a "windbag" or a short-tempered "bulldozer" or bully.

A woman wrote of a colleague during this exercise, "She is a lung dynamo. Like a whirlwind, she pulls in creative projects. She shouts: 'Do it! Change the world now.' A social committee of one, she has amazing creative and visionary insight into the next thing that needs to happen. As she blows onward, she leaves behind an 'It's good enough!' attitude, hoping a perfectionist will clean up after her."

A man complained about his sister who had held an important political office for years. "She always goes to the best hotels and orders the finest brandy for everyone. But," he complained, "she has lost herself. She knows what's best for her constituency, but not for herself. She and her assistants talk up every issue and work all hours. They are power mad."

Describe a situation in your life when you witnessed bullying or other dominating behavior.

Boasting. A physician who had studied the lungs on many levels described a man who went around telling others how to think and what to do. When he entered politics, he repeated his platform so often that at last his voters began to ask why he didn't follow through with what he said he would do. They invited him to a debate and tried every angle until they were exhausted with their efforts to get through to him. Tell a similar story with your own ending.

Wrestling with walls. Like the Indian widow described in this chapter in "The Story Behind the Sorrow," speak out a grievance that you have suppressed. Turn toward the four cardinal directions as you speak. Imagine the size, thickness, color, and age of the walls that tumble, and the new vistas opening before you as a result of the truth you speak.

Lungs and large intestine interviews. With a friend or colleague, take turns embodying the energies of the lungs and the large intestine by interviewing each other for a job. Imagine a lung-strong entrepreneur interviewing and recruiting a large-intestine-strong, detail-oriented person to carry out a big project. Write and perform this interview.

EXPANDING LUNG AWARENESS THROUGH DANCE, MUSIC, AND YOGA

Dance

With your thumbs up, imagine you are holding a big balloon in your hands. As you breathe deeply in and out, move your arms out and in as though the imaginary balloon is your lungs: the balloon filling and your arms opening out as you breathe in; the balloon deflating and your elbows coming in as you breathe out. Alternate contraction and expansion with your whole body as you crouch with bended knees, then prance and expand upward, trying to levitate like a magnificent balloon.

Music

Beethoven, *Ode to Joy*
Strauss, *Radetsky March*

Yoga asanas (Sanskrit names in italics)

Cat-Cow Stretch *(Bidalasana)*
Plank Pose *(Phalahakasana)*
Side Plank *(Vasisthasana)*
Push up *(Chaturanga)*
Handstand *(Muka Vrksasana)*

7

Catalyst: The Stomach

The word "stomach" derives from a Greek word *stoma,* meaning mouth. The whole alimentary tract, from taste buds and tongue to the supple and observant belly, is a prolonged mouth. The Old English word for this belly-mouth is *belg.* Our *belg* shrinks and swells according to our particular need and capacity. This magnificent tract, in which cosmic and earthly digestive forces have gathered over eons, eagerly incites us to seek what we need for greater well-being. Mental hunger and a spiritual nutritional process often accompany physical hunger. We may sometimes feel our whole being starving for greater love and for banquets of healing truth.

The stomach is located slightly to the left of the midline of the body, one of many subtle asymmetries that enliven us from within and exemplify the true meaning of "eccentric." A malleable little cooker, this very busy and ingenious organ seeks to balance itself and the whole body by hungrily summoning just the right food. The stomach is a sensitive distributing place that is constantly deciphering the exact needs of the body. It churns and processes spinach, bread, walnuts—whatever it has attracted to itself—striving with all its skill to transform foods to good use. Its smooth muscles agitate and mix. Meanwhile, acidic digestive juices arise from layers of uniquely responsive cells that work together in its lining. Chewed and swallowed food is transformed in the laboratories of the stomach and heated precisely. Because the stomach so skillfully combines foods for maximum energy, it also alerts the body when substances are not yet combined for optimal use. Preoccupied with receiving and breaking down food, stomach activity permeates every cell of the body, as each cell is sensitive to what it receives.

Acids in the stomach act ingeniously as catalytic agents and can send food back up and out with violent disgust, ecstatically savor, or go at digesting with plain diligence. The majority of us are born with digestive vigor and seldom notice the stomach's activities. Yet we can experience more consciously the stomach's resilient mode of service to the whole human body. Rub your stomach in a circle and pat your head quite vigorously at the same time. Then try reversing this by patting your stomach and rubbing your head. Alternate for a while. This will put a taste in your mouth for movement, and rouse you, heated and poised, for action. Gently swallow a few times and rub your stomach (just beneath your left rib cage). Let an energetic *m-m-m* fill your whole body with sensations of satisfying nourishment. Perhaps you will rouse from your vibrant stomach realm a buoyant tenor or contralto hum.

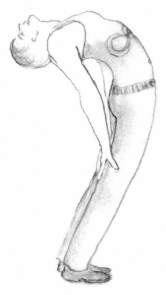

Stomach Exercise

As the healthy activity of the stomach produces a naturally positive attitude and lots of saliva, it wakes us up to the bounty of the natural world as we select and prepare our daily food. It wants us to sense the long journey of a carrot or apple from little seed, to behold in wonder cows being milked and butter being churned. It rejoices in a tasty row of lettuces and has us salivating at a ripening patch of raspberries.

As described by traditional Chinese medicine physicians, the stomach meridian begins next to the nose and makes a circuit around the mouth, eyes, ears, and temples. Then it moves down through the throat and the diaphragm to the stomach, descending through the abdomen and front of the thighs to above the second and third toes, finally emerging at the tips of the second toes.

Many people today lead sedentary lives. Confined at desks and in automobiles, very few of us sit upright. Muscular tensions build up in stomach and thighs. (A new trend even prevents children in public schools from playing outside during the schoolday.) Is it any wonder that an increasing number of people in every age category today have indigestion and sore legs?

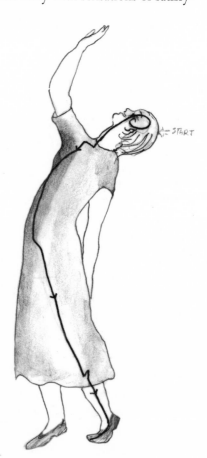

The Stomach Meridian

You can experience how tensions typically build up in stomach-based people by stretching and contracting the muscles at the front of your body. In a standing position, bend one knee and grasp the foot from behind. Contract your back muscles as you bend backward. Try to keep your thigh close to your other leg as you breathe. Then bend forward slightly, placing your free hand against a wall for balance. The quadriceps muscles at the front of your thigh will gradually lengthen. As you hold these openings and contractions, you will probably feel fascinating shifts. For example, with a powerful sense of anticipation, your body might propel forward. Hold the contraction even longer and a sense of fear and agitation might quite suddenly twist, and feel like an odd whirlybird or even a sudden fireworks display.

Tasting New Possibilities

I greatly admire strong-stomached people. They are invigorating, uninhibited catalysts and doers. Whether nimble physicians, gymnasts, or steeplejacks, they love challenges. They adapt to changing situations with a sense of adventure, and tend toward restless, foraging hyperactivity. Just as the stomach with its digestive enzymes naturally organizes food, strong-stomached folk tend to streamline jumbled complexities. Though they may often feel puzzled about themselves where their projects are concerned, they readily see how puzzling pieces fit into a larger picture. As they name and collate a turgid meal of impressions, they tend to generate new words and concepts to clarify and order their experiences. When the thought world connected with the stomach is thoroughly aroused, it can move at lightning speed, swiftly chewing through, digesting, and organizing an amazing amount of data.

Through their precise mental concepts, stomach people reach out and relate to others with inclusive organizing skills. They enjoy sharing their enthusiasms with all who come their way and quickly assimilate skills in whatever arena they turn to, whether gardening, skating, selling firecrackers, cooking, or managing an organic market. "Look at what I'm doing!" they exclaim, or "See what I discovered today!" As they draw a fascinated group around them to listen to their latest discoveries, they can astonish us, just as an exuberant burp honors a good meal in many cultures.

Anyone who has been truly hungry knows the sensation of life reviving in body and soul as soon as good food is circulating again. Highly effective stomach personalities can produce the sensation of enlivening nourishment. They can help whole groups of people simultaneously draw to them what is needed for their total well-being. Agile thinkers, they love to learn. Sharing their own thoughts without inhibition, they use flinty questions as firecrackers to dispel ignorance. They possess a natural, organic generosity and take a lively interest in how others are moving along with their lives. Team coaches with an optimistic outlook, they minutely observe, taking on and digesting difficulties with flashing intuition and gleeful bravado, quickly generating positives out of negatives, and getting on speedily with life.

People who live primarily oriented toward the stomach's activity naturally observe the physical, emotional, and spiritual effects of food. Like good physicians, they have enthusiasm for pinpointing remedies. A friend of mine with this discernment says, "Not that sweet muffin! You need fresh spinach and red onions in your system." Making very positive and precise suggestions, he knows exactly which food and medicinal substances are needed for anyone to function more fully. As he and similar folk satisfy their range of appetites, they resemble the stomach as it studies how to make food support the whole body. They rarely deprive themselves for long of what they need and enjoy.

A visit to a lively dance, yoga or exercise studio, or pool puts us in touch with these stomach people, young and old, who often feel compelled to explore the potential range of human motion. Highly sensitive to the need of every part of the body to receive proper nourishment and stimulation, stomach people encourage everyone to eat well and to exercise to their maximum, trying new and exciting twists and turns. They rejoice when others challenge themselves to bop and bustle and move more freely. They feel less alone as they constantly put themselves together like a puzzle through movement to ensure that every part of them is alive and well.

When I was a classroom teacher, an eight-year-old taught me a great deal about such superkinetic activity. He was a naturally happy, even euphoric boy. A bundle of electric energy, like other stomach sorts, his whole body would twist up like a pretzel when he was afraid of not doing a task well. One day, as his teacher, I went for a home visit. Insisting on my full attention, this adorable child actually scaled the wall of his bedroom to the angle where the wall met the ceiling. He hovered there for a few moments like a fly, and then tumbled back down onto his bed, bouncing for a while, humming with enthusiasm. Then he straightened himself up, and repeated his trick again and again. I wondered how I could possibly provide enough action for him in my classroom. He succeeded in inspiring much more rollicking lessons for the whole group than I had previously anticipated.

Busy "Red Hens"

As the busily brilliant minds of stomach-based people charge to meet daily challenges, their behavior can sometimes compare with an overly acidic stomach. Acidity affects the whole body and psyche. As stomach people go forward eagerly with their busy agendas, their expectations and ambitions may not have time to become grounded. Careening like whirlybirds toward more and more activity and less and less thought and reflection, they may lift off into their thought worlds, weakening the circuitry of energy that flows down into their legs and feet. If they are tired, they have a tendency to increase their activity. At the extreme, their kinesthetic and mental hyperactivity can resemble a high-voltage electrical storm or erratic fireworks, as menacing to themselves as to everyone around them. "Slow down!" we shout, as they ignore our pleas. Puzzling with ideas, striving to put all the pieces together, creating systems and theories, out of touch with themselves, only when they resume bodily observation do they come down to more sober reflections.

To healthy, active stomach types, everybody else can seem strangely, even frighteningly, lazy. Even when their inner weather system is calm, stomach personalities resemble the heroine of the English folktale "The Little Red Hen," as she busily goes about sowing, tending, and harvesting necessary food before winter. Like the stomach's kinesthetic coordination and nourishment of the total body, they seem to do most of the work. Capable of taking great care of a very complex realm, they strive to meet challenges with a quizzical smile and an undaunted attitude, and to make the best of any situation that comes their way.

A healthy stomach seeks to balance mind and body and create a natural high. Meeting one of these healthy stomachy people can be like finding a magical emerald. Ann Wigmore, who introduced the benefits of wheat grass and other "live foods" to the world, was just such a person. I volunteered for several years at the Ann Wigmore Foundation because I was so fascinated and inspired by her educational healing mission. A small, catalytic dynamo with saintly energy and devotion, she changed my life. True to the stomach's mission, Ann catalyzed new consciousness for my total well-being. Millions of people and animals have benefited from her journey of self-healing, which is recounted in her autobiography, entitled *Why Suffer?*

COMMUNICATING WITH THE STOMACH

Like all of our organs, the stomach gradually learns to regulate its rhythmic activities and to adjust to the food that is available. Especially in childhood and adolescence, the stomach can seem to take over in the body. Without adult guidance, it can wreak havoc. Hard-pressed to balance emotional and physical demands, its sometimes wild appetites have inspired countless stories to delight children, such as this Russian version of "The Gingerbread Boy.

⁕⁕⁕⁕⁕

The Clay Pot Boy

One day a childless old man and woman decided to take some clay and carefully make a version of a boy. They baked him in the oven. When they took him out, much to their surprise, the boy looked at them both and said, "I'm hungry. Give me something to eat." So the old man and the old woman brought him all they had—bread and jam, pickles and ham, and mustard sauce—but it wasn't enough. He said, "I still want more."

"Well, there is no more," said the old couple.

So the boy opened his mouth and ate the old man and the old woman. Then he walked down the road until he met a rooster and he said, "I've eaten my father, I've eaten my mother, I ate the bread, I ate the jam, the pickles and ham, and mustard sauce, and I still want more."

"Well, there is no more," said the rooster. So the boy opened his mouth and ate the rooster, and walked on down the road until he met a pig, a cow, a barn full of chickens and all their eggs.

At last he met a billy goat, and the billy goat said, "Well, you're not going to eat me." He butted the clay pot boy with his horns, and the clay pot boy broke in two. Out came the barn full of chickens with all their eggs, the cow, the pig, the rooster, the old woman, the old man, the bread, the jam, the pickles, the ham, and last but not least, the mustard sauce, of course.

⊱•✽•⊰

The regurgitation at the end of this story gives a merciful sense of relief, and inspires us to seek more delightful ways to experience comfort and well-being than by overeating.

The belly is particularly responsive to musical tones. Parents often discover that humming soothes ruffled children. As the parents hum, croon, and share a story that addresses the stomach realm, their children can fully relax. My elderly aunt once discovered that a tiny expressive mouse had somehow found its way into her warm bed in the middle of the night. The mouse was singing a duet back and forth with her stomach, which was rumbling loudly because of the large salad she had eaten for dinner. Can we, too, learn to communicate directly with our stomachs?

A learned man joined one of my storytelling circles to see if making a story himself would help him in his voracious appetite for books and food. Like the Clay Pot Boy, his stomach seemed to be jammed wide open. In his childhood, he had very dutifully lost all sense of proportion as he tried to please his parents by overeating their food and by compulsive academic achievement. He could eat a whole pie and consume ten books after dinner. One evening during the course, after much resistance, his imagination delivered to him just the story he needed to hear. As he spoke, he let himself exaggerate his plight in a heart-rending and frightening short tale about a man who got on a train and then ate everything in it, including the passengers. At last the man in his story ate the train too. After this mythic binge, however, the story took a turn for the better. His protagonist discovered a beautiful child toddling toward him over a green hill. When his story was finished, he sat still for a long time, feeling unconditional love for his very real young daughter, and hers for him. He breathed a huge sigh of relief and quietly shed tears of joy. Like many other people, he had discovered with luminous insight the satisfying sense of love that arises independent of food and mental achievement.

Storytellers throughout time have explored themes of too much and too little, of glut and famine. Robin Williamson, the great Scots storyteller, retells a rollicking tale called "The Vision of MacConglinne" that was first written down in the twelfth century. This rhymed tale tells of a king who was afflicted with a terrible "unnatural craving for comestibles and potations."

At last the renowned poet MacConglinne came to his rescue. With great charm and ingenuity, he presented the king with a challenge to rid him of his obsession with food. "Fast with me until morning," said the poet, and the king agreed.

All that night they rested, and at the first light of day MacConglinne ordered fires to be kindled and cooks to cook. But he also ordered manacles and chains, with which the king was securely fastened. Then the poet began to dip morsels in honey and to wave them in front of the king's nose, at which the king writhed and roared. A guard passed in front of him with every imaginable delectable dish. All the while the poet tempted and teased him, reciting wild gastronomic visions in delicious rhyme. At last, he chanted a powerful spell:

> Go now in the name of Cheese,
> and may Bacon guard you,
> and Yellow Thick Cream preserve you,
> and the Mighty Cauldron of Soup watch over you.

And as MacConglinne was saying these words, the demon imp of hunger who had come to live in the poor afflicted king showed its sleek dark face in the king's gaping mouth. Trying to reach all the real and imaginary food, the imp leaned out from the king's mouth farther…and farther…until at last it fell with a terrible yell into the heart of the fire, and the king was cured.

Another overeating story originates from the Benin tribe of Nigeria.

⌘⌘⌘⌘⌘

Eating the Sky

There was a time when no one who lived on Earth had to work because the sky provided everything. If the people were hungry, they had only to reach up and they received exactly what they needed.

Sometimes, however, people would break off more than they could chew, and what they didn't want they cast aside. That was easy for the people, but the sky didn't like seeing itself treated like rubbish. One day it spoke out: "People, if you go on wasting what I give to you, I will do something you will regret."

For a while the people remembered what the sky said and no one took more than they really needed. But one day a greedy fellow who always liked more than enough grabbed a piece of sky big enough to feed himself, his family, and his friends for weeks. He chomped and swallowed what he could, threw the rest down, and walked away.

The sky was silent was a while, and then it let out a roar and rose up and up, and it went on rising. When the people saw what had happened, they came running out of their houses, crying, "Come back. Please come back!" But the sky was out of reach by then. The next morning the people were hungry, and the next day hungrier still. They had to till the ground and grow some food, and that is why we all have been working ever since.

⌘

STARVATION SPEAKS

When people know what it is to be famished, sometimes over long years, their suffering can stimulate another sort of story. A middle-European folktale among those collected by the Brothers Grimm tells of a starving child and her mother.

⌘

Sweet Porridge

The hungry child went into the forest. There an aged woman who was aware of her sorrow met her and presented her with a little pot, which would cook good, sweet porridge when she said, "Cook, little pot, cook," and would cease to cook when she said, "Stop, little pot." The child took the pot home and she and her mother were freed from their poverty and hunger, and ate sweet porridge as often as they chose. Once when the child had gone out, the mother said, "Cook, little pot, cook." And it did cook and she ate till she was satisfied. Then she wanted the pot to stop cooking but did not know what to say. So the little pot went on cooking and the porridge rose over the edge, and still it cooked on until the kitchen and whole house were full, and the next house, and then the whole street, just as if it wanted to satisfy the hunger of the whole world. But no one knew how to stop it. At last when only one house remained visible, the child came home and just said, "Stop, little pot," and it stopped and gave up cooking, and those who wished to return to the town had to eat their way back.

⌘

IN SEARCH OF BALANCE

A woman who grew up with many problems related to eating and digesting food participated in my "Storytelling as a Healing Art" course. She had been a successful nutritional counselor for several years, and had chosen this profession out of her strong desire to help both herself and others find a healthy relationship with food. "My patients are a patchwork of what modern people have to deal with. I have a mission to help them build and repair their damaged appetite for life," she said. "This work feeds my compassion." During one of the group sessions, she told us how her hysterically busy mother had judged her on her appearance and given her very little warmth and acceptance. She sensed that being rejected had turned into the belly cramps that decreased the flow of acids and enzymes in her stomach. Like many people with her dynamic sensitivities, as a young woman she was bulimic and suffered from a painful duodenal ulcer.

During the course, the story she created came to her like a healing dream. Later she performed it for us. Casting her struggles into a strange tale and presenting it as a "one-woman show" helped her to digest the excruciating self-consciousness she had experienced as a child. As she caricatured her feelings, she was able to experience them more freely and clearly. She called her story "Young Woman with a Showcase."

Once there was a young woman who was born with a strange condition. Instead of flesh and blood, her middle body was a glass showcase. She grew up feeling different in a circus, surrounded by many talented acrobats and trapeze artists. It was a very busy and always colorful buzzing world amongst all these circus people.

On her thirteenth birthday, the girl decided to run away. She ran and ran without knowing where to go or where to stop, until she came to a small village with an open market square. She decided to stand next to the church and display her showcase, hoping she would be able to earn some money in this way.

Visitors queued up in long meandering lines to stare into this unusual showcase. She would not speak, nor would she move. Little flames would creep over her skin, turning it bright red. Only when each visitor had turned his back to the showcase would her skin calm down.

One evening a big storm was gathering in the sky. The clouds became bigger and bigger and hung very low, and when the wind had built up into a hefty gale, it took the young woman into the air and blew her right up into a tree.

One of the big branches pierced her right through the middle and her showcase broke into a thousand little pieces. Shattered glass and the broken pieces of many showcase objects rained down. The wind took them and spread them over the land.

The young woman was in excruciating pain. At last the tree could not bear listening to her screaming any longer and asked the gray-feathered birds usually resting on its branches to help. So the birds let some of their feathers fall down and the tree shook and loosened the petals of its pink and white blossoms. And while they were falling, the feathers and the petals started to weave a tissue, a very delicate white silky fabric. Feathers and petals gave it density and flexibility, and the tissue grew stronger.

At last the tree swayed to release the young woman onto the ground. As she stood on her feet again, the newly woven loveliness wrapped around her middle and attached itself to her hips and just under her breasts. The young woman was astonished. She cautiously touched herself, and as she stroked, she noticed that her midriff took on the appearance of ordinary skin, with veins and blood and flesh, like anybody else's. Later, as she went out into the world, whenever she saw a tree swaying with the melody of the wind, or birds flying in the blue sky, she would smile with a deep sense of gratitude and awe.

After her performance, the woman wrote, "Writing and performing the story brought me down out of my head into a creative digestive flow. I could feel the story working through my negativity. While standing in front of the whole group to tell this story aloud, I really enjoyed expressing exactly what I feel. I think this story is partly about the creative side of my psyche wanting to grow and fully *stomach* my life.

TRANSFORMATIONAL STORYTELLING

Stomach Affirmation
I create catalytic movement for the benefit of all.

Basic Stomach Story Dynamic
Addiction turns into brilliant feeding of self and others.

Stomach Protagonists and Antagonists
Stomach protagonists (characters who support stomach health) are candid and conversational. Constantly thinking of how to advance goals and fulfill wishes, they encourage others to express themselves without inhibition. They are optimistic, future-minded, interdisciplinary, and purposeful thinkers and organizers of information. Exuberant workers and innovators with great perseverance, they hone in on the exceptional uniqueness of individuals, places, things, and food.

Stomach antagonists (characters who express stomach dysfunction) are greedy for food and quick "fixes." Confused and mentally tormented by pervasive physical and mental distress, they tend toward verbal aggression. Oblivious of social norms, they are maverick and dilettantish, with poor judgment about themselves and others.

Basic Story Elements
Myths and stories often resonate with specific internal processes. This reliable pattern invokes well-being and resilience in every cell of your body:

Setting Out: The protagonist sets out in quest of greater love, strength, justice, wisdom, and happiness.

Trouble: One or more obstacles and/or antagonists interfere with the journey.

Help: Wise and benevolent help comes, often giving a gift.

Positive Ending: The protagonist fulfils the quest with joy and celebration.

SUMMONING YOUR STORYTELLER

Stomach-dominant storytellers tell stories as much through movement and audience response as through speaking. They share the latest dynamic episode of their lives, gesturing with their whole bodies. Uninhibited and subversive in expression, they naturally expose what others deny. With an ear for colloquialisms, they do not shy away from being shocking. They dress for comfort and freedom of movement, and enjoy sharing stories that require their audiences to get up and move, such as "Joe and the Button Factory" (see following). They want others to become more aware of how they live in their bodies and lives altogether, and to awaken new flexibility and clarity.

Exercises to Explore and Balance the Stomach

Creating characters to balance the stomach. Make up a story about a character, or perhaps a whole tribe, that is troubled by one or more of the antagonist's characteristics listed. Like Aladdin with his magic lamp, a healthy stomach gains energy from challenge. Let both body and soul be fed as your protagonist moves toward satisfying fulfillment.

Blasting off with cannons and fireworks. To feel the bells-and-whistles intensity of a stomach hero or heroine, listen to the finale of Tchaikovsky's *1812 Overture*. Rub your belly until its hums and, with the help of your inner storyteller, create such a protagonist. When stories create arenas of health and safety, they are ultimately relaxing and fun. Now create a character or two to embody the stomach's shadow realm. Perhaps your characters long for a food binge or other quick fix. They might start eating themselves by biting their lips and tongue. Oblivious of social norms, they might be verbally aggressive oddballs with poor judgment about themselves and others. To experience a healing dynamic, continue the story. Your stomachy protagonist possesses delightful mythic power to advance goals and fulfill wishes. What happens as your antagonist and protagonist meet? Let the plot evolve until the virtues of the stomach prevail over its shadow realm.

Let a different protagonist set out on a journey toward a place of "m-m-m" deliciousness, connectedness, and satisfaction. Let this protagonist soon encounter opposition. The obstacle zone might be connected with a real problem in your own life or the life of someone close to you. A bothersome hyperactive person in your life might be portrayed as an old woman in the market who does not stop talking and pretends to have done what she has not accomplished, or perhaps a wizard who distracts with difficult and mesmerizing puzzles that cannot be solved. Then a helping force comes—and to end, a satisfying feast.

Wishes, food, and biography. Have you been fed love and appreciation today? What does your stomach desire now to truly nourish you, body and soul? Sit back and, through the power of your imagination, call a genie to provide just that on a golden platter.

Favorite memories of food make wonderful stories. A friend of mine helps people tell their biographies by focusing on the whole long history of their relationship with food. Her therapy sessions often take place in her wonderfully colorful kitchen. Describe the very first meal you can remember. Describe in detail at least one of your favorite, most nourishing meals.

Movement stories. Go into nature, observe carefully, and dance what you see. Tell "Eating the Sky," the earlier story from Nigeria, purely in movement, or invite your listeners to move the story as you tell it aloud.

Joe and the button factory. The purpose of this story is to get into motion. Try telling this silly story aloud to others, keeping the same gestures for each phrase that repeats.

Hello, my name is Joe and I work in a button factory
I have a house, and a dog, and a family
One day, my boss said to me, "Hey, Joe, are you busy?"
I said, "No."
"Then turn the button with your left hand."

Hello, my name is Joe and I work in a button factory
I have a house, and a dog, and a family
One day, my boss said to me, "Hey, Joe, are you busy?"
I said, "No."
"Then turn the button with your right hand."

Hello, my name is Joe and I work in a button factory
I have a house, and a dog, and a family
One day, my boss said to me, "Hey, Joe, are you busy?"
I said, "No."
"Then turn the button with your left foot."

Hello, my name is Joe and I work in a button factory
I have a house, and a dog, and a family
One day, my boss said to me, "Hey, Joe, are you busy?"
I said, "No."
"Then turn the button with your right foot."

Hello, my name is Joe and I work (real hard) in a button factory
I have a house, and a dog, and a family
One day, my boss said to me, "Hey, Joe, are you busy?"
I said, "No."
"Then turn the button with your head."

Hello, my name is Joe and I work in a button factory
I have a house, and a dog, and a family
One day, my boss said to me, "Hey, Joe, are you busy?"
I said, "Yes!"

Expanding Stomach Awareness Through Dance, Music, and Yoga

Dance

Place your hands on the small of your back, keeping your feet shoulder-width apart. Gently loosen your jaw and tongue, and look up. Release your shoulders back and downward as you lift your torso upward. Bending slightly backward, move from your belly in as many directions as you can find. Opening and closing your jaw, feel your whole digestive tract opening and closing, too, mobilizing every part of your body. Imagine that you are digesting a delicious feast as you move freely about the room.

Music

Rossini, *William Tell* Overture
Bach, *Violin Concerto in E Major,* the first movement
Satie, *La Belle Excentrique* and *Les Aventures de Mercure*
Vivaldi, Spring from *The Four Seasons*

Yoga asanas (Sanskrit names in italics)

Awkward *(Utkatasana)*
Camel *(Ustrasana)*
Bow *(Dhanurasana)*
Stomach-releasing *(Supta-Vajrasana)*

8

Peaceful Protectors:
The Spleen and the Pancreas

The spleen is a mysterious lymphatic organ, located just beneath the heart. This crucial organ receives and cradles new blood, gently swaying it onward toward wider circulation. It is a training center for immune cells and the lively meeting place where our blood gathers to develop its individual stamp of resilience. Esoteric traditions describe the spleen as our inner Saturn, the mighty protector and harmonizer of the whole body's inner planets and stars, the guardian of the threshold between cosmic influences and human individuality. Rudolf Steiner called the spleen "the most spiritual of organs." Swaying slightly while reading or reciting scripture or listening to music activates its spiritual wings. As familiar conventional Earth boundaries fade, the physically based self begins to sense the vast processes internalized in our spleen and pancreas, as in all our physical organs.

Adjacent to the spleen, just above and behind the stomach, lives the pancreas. The pancreas is the guardian of sweetness for the whole body. Whereas salt furrows a brow and brings on earthly concerns, sweetness softly expands into childlike spacious rapture. Its daily work is the creation, digestion, and circulation of various kinds of sweetness throughout the whole system. The lattice-like wing of delicate fibers that holds this long narrow organ in place resembles other lymph nodes scattered throughout the body. As the body continuously seeks balance, the pancreas secretes insulin and glycogen, hormones that regulate blood sugar. It also secretes pancreatic juices into the duodenum that help digest proteins, fats, and starches.

In traditional Chinese medicine, the activities of the spleen and pancreas are linked in one meridian that originates on the inner side of the big toes. As these energies support our well-being, they ascend the inner ankles and continue upward through the torso to the throat, ending at the root on the underside of the tongue. A branch of this spleen meridian moves through the pancreas to the heart, where it connects with the heart meridian. The Chinese, who treat chronic bleeding diseases through the spleen meridian, see it as a secondary womb from which fresh new life springs. Guardian of the body's ever-renewing blood supply, it rules the sense of purity throughout our whole being. It sends energy to the lungs where blood and breath meet. Muscle tone throughout the body can indicate its relative strength or weakness.

EXPERIENCING SPLEEN AND PANCREAS ENERGY

Sway while softly pursing your lips. What do you feel? Now lift your arms gently like wings or sails unfurling to the wind. Let your forefingers first touch lightly above your head and then waft them down to meet behind you at the base of your spine. As many children discover spontaneously in their dreams, or lying with arms outstretched in the snow, the full mystery of the human form includes a span of invisible wings. These possess an intelligence of their own. Let your shoulders and back muscles soften. Imagine yourself with ethereal wings moving freely through space, like the Greek messenger Nike. As when children play together, you may feel heavenly laughter from an unknown source surrounding you and bubbling up within you.

Sweetness creates an expansive relationship with space. The freshness of love or childbirth, or perhaps of tasting chocolate and fine wine, gives hints of how, beyond our usual sense of measured space and time, we are composed of invisible forces and wholly connected with higher realms. However solid we may feel, we may suddenly open to these mysterious dimensions. Where do we come from, and where are we going as part of the teeming universe? As our spiritual awareness expands, the human body and all of the natural world enlarges into more spacious dimensions. From the impulses that pour through the spleen and pancreas, a sense of spiritual protection manifests throughout the world. Images of physical-spiritual beings abound in cathedrals, Hindu and Buddhist temples, and Chinese paintings. They throng in the spirited works of William Blake and Marc Chagall.

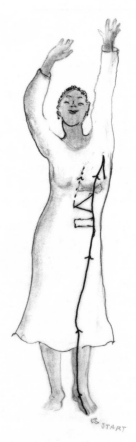

The Spleen-Pancreas Meridian

Spiritual expansion requires new maps. When I first began practicing yoga stretches that connect with the spleen meridian at Bob Cooley's Boston Meridian Stretching Center, I experienced surprising and somewhat disconcerting expansions. I felt that I might easily fly through windows and walls and join church bells and birds soaring over the rooftops of Boston. I continued strengthening the spleen-pancreas meridian through stretching exercises at home. Early one morning, I was astonished to feel the universe pouring into me. I was surprised to see a small blue light shining within my forehead. Soon afterward, I became aware of the whole Earth as a small blue orb in measureless space, surrounded by a vast network of protective presences. I sensed these presences to be weaving and working together, forming a soft blue halo around the Earth. Until then I had merely believed in the possibility of angels. Feeling completely astonished and with a profound sense of protection, as I settled down from this truly spiritual experience, scenes played in my mind from *Wings of Desire,* a film that portrays human souls who died in war-torn Germany and return as angels to fly freely to those who need them. I remembered how Jonathan Livingston Seagull flew through walls, and how certain Western and Eastern saints have learned how to live entirely on spiritual nourishment.

LIVING THE BLESSED LIFE

Anyone who has followed a cleansing regimen soon realizes that healthy clean blood influences every aspect of our lives. It clears murky feelings and thoughts and opens doors and windows to the spiritual dimensions of life. It moistens and reddens tongue and lips. Spleen activity makes it possible for the vibratory rhythms in food substances to adapt to individual needs. If the spleen is weak, the lips are pale and the mouth becomes insensitive to taste. Healthy spleen people are very aware of whatever touches their lips. They are excellent caterers and providers of whole foods and spices. Because they seek a sense of balance and lightness from food, and from all their activities, they naturally insist on purity; they are careful how they combine different foods so as not to burden their digestive system. They fast to feel fresh and clean, and tend to organize their meals carefully for balance and purity. They may eat often and slowly, and experiment with unusual diets—for the fun of it, and because they are so sensitive to the effects of food and drink. While they can seem to others to invent food fads and be obsessed with obtaining the right food to the detriment of their other needs, they often inspire others to be more aware of the polluting effects of food and environment. At best, they improve the diets of others as they tend their own. Their occasional coconut angel food cake can taste especially heavenly.

In direct contrast with the digestive fireworks of the stomach personality, there is a kind of ineffable bounce about those who inhabit the energies of the spleen and pancreas. Living lightly between matter and spirit, a luminosity arises from within them. They easily accept, and easily give. With abundant and amiable sheltering impulses, they are natural caretakers. Purifying and uplifting, their presence brings a relaxed feeling of safety to others, and similar nurturing to the surrounding landscape. They raise butterflies, build bird sanctuaries, and purvey subtle flower essences and homeopathic medicines. As midwives, they bring joy and safety to the threshold of birth. As hospice workers, they ease death. A story or a conversation with them can feel like a boat floating on a pleasantly flowing river. They are expansive songsters and writers through whom words flow freely, giving a refreshing sense of the swing and sway of life.

ANGELS IN OUR MIDST

Like many counselors and others who strive to transform food and drug addiction in communities, Tom is a young man whose personality reflects the work of the spleen and pancreas. Having overcome his own addictions, he has become an effective drug counselor who coaxes people away from substances that harm their bodies and their total well-being. Around him glows a deliciously soft atmosphere. Even as he works hard, he purses his lips and often hums to concentrate. He gives the impression of freshness, like a child imbued with sweetness and light. As he works at his desk, his big toes pressing down, he gently sways back and forth, pausing easily to answer the telephone. With congenial openness, he smiles and gently leans to embrace each newcomer to his office.

How do spleen and pancreas–dominant people become so accessible and light, so luminously fun-loving? As they tend to locate their awareness outside their physical bodies, they inspire us to loosen our relationship with gravity and with time and space. Around them walls disappear. At a party, they offer exquisitely soft kisses and embraces instead of bone-cracking hugs and handshakes. They surround and protect, offering guidance and sharing the best information about how to feel good and to have good times. Though they may seem forgetful and vague at times, the fresh blood that radiates through their whole being allows them to merge easily with others, creating pleasantly uplifting and calming encounters.

For Fran and Mickey, a spleen-strong couple, money and possessions move lightly. Just for the fun of it, they often rearrange the heavy furniture in their house and garden. As a pastime, Fran makes little angels out of lamb's wool and gives them away wherever she goes with her young children, even to the bankteller and grocer. In the wee hours of the morning, she sometimes paints multitudes of angels weaving together in multidimensional space, their gazes turning in every direction. Taking her work lightly, one day she wrapped and tied several of her paintings around some trees. She suspended other angelic creations with clothespins in her outdoor gallery. Another day she forgot she had hung a big painting that she had worked on for years on a garage door. When by mistake the automatic garage door opened, the painting went flying. "It was fun," she said without dismay. "I let it go." A well-known adage says: "Angels fly because they take themselves lightly."

Spleen and pancreas–dominant folk usually have an affinity with the "sweet life" and prefer to relax and enjoy. They have the knack of working primarily to feel good and to have fun. Even in the midst of very challenging projects, they carry an uncanny mood that reminds us of the places we want to go for paradisal holidays. At political gatherings, they may show up wearing party clothes. Mirroring the expansive and regulatory roles of pancreas and spleen, whether nurses or environmentalists, playful kindergarten teachers, painters of spiritual landscapes, florists, or flutists, their subtle energy acts as a purifying system to the whole body and psyche. As colonic therapists, they pleasantly share useful health information as they wash people free of unhealthy intestinal accumulations. With serenity and joy, they devote themselves to singing and dancing to bring about peace. Their prayers can cause communal enjoyment as they help everyone push through the past with its guilt and blame, and open the way to the ineffable grandeur of the present moment. They "channel" messages from on high.

People whose lives radiate an atmosphere of sweetness and light sometimes enjoy having saltier folk to sober them. When they find themselves arriving late for appointments, wearing a saccharine smile, perhaps with something important left unspoken, they gravitate toward more straightforward folk who bring them solidly down to Earth.

COMING DOWN TO EARTH

The English storyteller Pat Bowen tells a folksy, irreverent story about three angels who wanted to have nothing to do with Earth. This was because they looked down and saw people getting drunk, abusing sexuality, and killing each other. The angels felt that Earth was a place they should never go.

Angels are as numerous as blades of grass, yet it took a long time for God to convince three of them to experience Earth for themselves. These three agreed, but only on condition that they would have nothing to do with drunkenness, sexual excess, or murder. They descended, dressed themselves as humans, and walked about on Earth, listening to human conversations and watching what was going on. They were totally disgusted.

Soon, however, a woman happened to notice the glorious visitors and, with an irresistible wink, invited them to her place. The angels could not say no. She prepared a magnificent feast for them. Peach juice dribbled down their chins, they began to taste fine wine on their tongues, and it wasn't long before they were completely drunk. She took care of them, as she was that sort of woman, and they had a wild time. You can imagine. The angels were having such a wild time that a man passing by looked over the wall to see what was going on. It was then that one of the angels picked up a bottle and hurled it—and killed him.

Then the angels realized they had broken their three golden rules. Mortified, they remembered the secret mantras they had been given that would return them to the divine world. These they quickly spoke, and whoosh, they were transported again to the throne of God. There they fell on their faces, absolutely filled with shame. But God smiled, saying: "Now you know it is not easy for human beings." The woman had heard the mantra and when she too arrived in heaven, God lifted her into the sky to shine as a beacon.

PEACE AND RECONCILIATION

Frans Koenigs, a Dutch storyteller and peace advocate who works with war veterans, wrote the following story during a healing story course. He intentionally wrote the story to reflect the physiological dynamics of his most familiar zone of body and soul: the pancreas and spleen. Writing the story brought him to a new level of understanding of his desire to heal violence.

～～～～～

When I Was a Little Lamb

I want to take you to the time I was a little lamb. I will start by making an odd noise: Mtja Mtja Mtja. May I ask you to join me in making that sound together? Mtja, mtja, oh, this sweet sound! It is the sound we sheep make when we are eating together. For me it is the sound of peace and togetherness and safety. We were so proud to be sheep at that time. We felt ourselves the alpha and omega of life. The peace we created together radiated far beyond the meadow. On Earth, we were the gentle breath of heaven.

Right from the beginning of being a lamb, I loved to wander out alone to the edges of the meadow. I loved to be close to the water at sunset. Our shadows would become long and the grass inside the shadows would become purple. We are eating the grass of our shadows, I used to think. But then my mother would call me with her sweet voice, and I would recognize her voice from a thousand others because my mother had the sweetest voice of them all. And I would run toward her, straight against the light of the setting sun, which would blind me. My feet would hardly touch the ground, and I would feel completely light and happy. If you were to ask me to picture happiness, it would be this: me running toward my mother, with the light of the sun in my face. I would bump my head against her udder and the sweetest, creamiest milk you ever tasted would spring forth—life itself. That is how happy life was, until there was a rumor about wolves…

It happened that I was still a young and small lamb when the wolves, clever as they are, caught me and ate me. Then I was part of a wolf. Eventually, I was reborn as a little wolf, and I learned how intelligently they run their society and raise their little ones. I loved bounding over the fields and stalking prey at the edge of the forest, and especially I loved gathering with my fellow wolves and howling. That was the best of all.

Then a farmer shot me, and the next thing I knew I was a human child who loved his pet dog and dreamed of growing up to be a soldier carrying a gun and killing enemies. And so this too came to pass.

I soon found out that being a soldier and carrying a gun was not fun. I did not like to shoot the gun. One day I became separated from my regiment. I came to a river and I was confused. Perhaps I was wounded, perhaps even dead. It must have been my spirit that saw the blood-filled ocean. For in time, I was flying above it, looking down over children, women, men, and animals, their faces filled with despair. I looked into one pair of eyes and then into the next and the next. I went from one face to another for long lifetimes. There was no face, however broken or tortured, that I didn't look at. And after a long time, something within me began to change. I found peace as great as the universe.

⥹⥹⥹⥹⥹

Writing and telling his story has helped Frans develop his work. He often tells his visionary tale to open his workshops with war veterans and young people who have suffered violent experiences. By connecting deeply with the soul-spiritual processes within his own body, he is able to help others to experience from within themselves how violently destructive impulses carried in the blood can transform into a peaceful life stream.

WINGED BEINGS AS BELOVED COMPANIONS

Blocked spiritual life can result in unhappiness and diseases of the blood and digestion. As the health of the spleen diminishes, we might feel amorphous and unreliable, our bones and vision growing weaker. Fatty deposits and florid skin eruptions might disturb us. Depressed immune function in the spleen impacts the whole body and soul. We may feel incapable of doing what we say, and not follow through. Exhausted from self-sacrificing and suffering, a hole may seem to open in the universe. Instead of experiencing angels, instead some may even feel or see weirdly splenetic demons. Many legends and fairytales assure us that, even in our darkest moments, immensely benevolent spiritual companionship is near to support us. The Book of Tobit is one of the books of the Apocrypha not included in many standard versions of the Old Testament.

⥹⥹⥹⥹⥹

Tobias and the Angel

Tobit, a just man, lived with his good wife, Anna, caring for the dying and ensuring that they received proper burial. Yet one day sparrows let fall their droppings into old Tobit's eyes and blinded him. Unable then to continue his good works, he called his son Tobias to him, and said, "I would like you to collect some money that is owed to me by my kinsman in Media. It shall be your inheritance. Find someone to show you the way."

Not long thereafter, young Tobias met a man who was familiar with all the highways and byways on the route, and offered to accompany him on his journey. Tobit and Anna approved of this guide and companion, so they all said their farewells and the two set out on the long journey, Tobias's little white dog at their heels.

They came in the evening to the River Tigris. Tobias had taken off his shoes to wash his feet when a mighty fish leapt out of the river. Then his companion said to Tobias, "Take the fish and remove the heart, the liver, and the gallbladder. Keep these safe." The two of them then ate what remained of the fish and were satisfied.

After a long journey, they arrived at the house of Raguel, a relative of Tobias, and were met by the daughter, a beautiful young woman named Sarah, who was Tobias's cousin. The two of them fell in love and wished to be married. A great darkness hung over the household, however. Sarah had been married seven times before, and each time on her wedding night, her husband had died. Her father was deeply concerned that this would happen again.

It was then that Tobias's companion advised him: "Those who succumb to evil enter marriage without gratitude to God. Spend three days in prayer. On your wedding night, be with Sarah, burn the fish's heart and liver as incense on burning coals. The fumes will drive away the evil spirit that caused the deaths of her previous husbands."

The father of the house knew Sarah would make his nephew a fitting wife and he, too, was assured by Tobias's traveling companion. So the two young people entered the wedding chamber, and Tobias did as his companion had advised him to do. The evil spirit tried to creep into the room but was soon repulsed by the fumes of incense from the burning heart and liver. It fled into the desert, never to return.

Thus the lovers survived the night. But that was not the end of the blessings. Two weeks of great festivities followed in celebration of their wedding, with singing and dancing. Tobias received the money that was owed. Then with his wife and his companion, he returned home with great rejoicing to his blinded father. Seeing the suffering of the old man, Tobias's companion said, "Place the gall of the fish on the eyes of your father." When Tobias had done this, Tobit was healed and could see, and again there was great singing and dancing.

"What will you do for your companion?" old Tobit asked his son. "He showed you the way, saved your life, and made sure that you received your inheritance. How can we ever repay him?"

Then the companion blazed with the splendor of his true being: "I am Raphael. I ask for no recompense. I was sent by God so that Tobias might fulfill his destiny."

All the wedding guests immediately fell on their faces and Raphael, as quietly and invisibly as he had come, went on his way.

⁓⁓⁓

Like the spleen itself, the angel was in touch with the healing majesty of the heart, liver, and gall. He guided their contributions to the well-being of Tobias and his extended family. Winged beings abound as helpers to mythic and literary heroes and heroines. The Greeks pictured the god Hermes as a young man with the first down on his cheeks, flying through their poetry and song with wings on his staff, cap, and sandals, guiding and offering protection. Ariel, the nature spirit in Shakespeare's play *The Tempest,* helped the great magician Prospero fulfill his destiny.

The Oil of Mercy

A compilation of sacred texts called *The Golden Legend* tells of Seth, the third son of Adam and Eve. Adam had already lived for 923 years in the Hebron valley when he realized that at last it was time for him to die. He longed to reconcile the murderous relationship between Cain and Abel, Seth's brothers. So he sent Seth to the gate of Paradise to beg for the Oil of Mercy.

Seth set out for the Paradise that his parents had known before they resigned themselves to an earthly mortal life. When he arrived on his errand of mercy for his dying father, he met an angel who gave him the sacred oil of heavenly compassion. The angel also gave him three seeds from the original Tree of Life. Seth returned the long way home to Earth, and blessed and anointed his old father with this oil. Then he placed the three seeds under Adam's tongue. It is said that from these three seeds, and from Adam's holy body, grew the tree that later bore the body of Christ into Paradise.

Much traditional iconography expresses the power of resurrection that on a smaller scale plays out in the spleen every day, lifting consciousness so that more than earthly powers may germinate, root, and grow within us. So it was that in the biblical account of the life of Jacob, the founder of Israel, in Genesis 32, Jacob ferried his family to safety across a stream, returning to the other side alone to retrieve "small jars." During his long dark night there alone, he was awakened to wrestle with an unknown angel until dawn. At daybreak, injured but not defeated, he held his combatant, saying, "I will not let you go until you bless me." The angel indeed blessed him, and so through Jacob a new people sprang, with a bloodline of unfathomable resilience. Thus the truth that pours into all humanity insists that though we suffer untold bodily harm, spiritual anguish, and darkness, when we insist on a blessing, great spiritual gifts of resilience and joy can be won.

As the morning light gathers, the spleen awakens to serve the whole body. As these subtle radiations of spleen energy gather and rise, they encourage a tendency to willing sacrifice. The sublime end point of the spleen and pancreas meridian's rising energy just under the tongue can have the effect of a sacramental wafer, and of sublime spiritual nectar. Its natural crown of energy produced in the head can feel like a halo or, conversely, like a crown of thorns.

TRANSFORMATIONAL STORYTELLING

Spleen and Pancreas Affirmation

I find within me the purity and sweetness I seek.

Basic Spleen and Pancreas Story Dynamic

Codependency becomes conscious empathy.

Spleen and Pancreas Protagonists and Antagonists

Spleen and pancreas protagonists (characters who support spleen and pancreas health) are peacemakers, empathetic, interdependent, patient, and diplomatic. They nurture contented relationships and focus on the good of all.

Spleen and pancreas antagonists (characters who express spleen and pancreas dysfunction) are sugary and superficial, pleasing and ineffectual. With mental confusion, worries, and boredom, they spend their time trying to be excessively helpful to others. They sacrifice themselves while bringing others down with them, serving no one.

Basic Story Elements

Myths and stories often resonate with specific internal processes. This reliable pattern invokes well-being and resilience in every cell of your body:

Setting Out: The protagonist sets out in quest of greater love, strength, justice, wisdom, and happiness.

Trouble: One or more obstacles and/or antagonists interfere with the journey.

Help: Wise and benevolent help comes, often giving a gift.

Positive Ending: The protagonist fulfils the quest with joy and celebration.

SUMMONING YOUR STORYTELLER

Storytellers with dominant spleen-pancreas energy often feel themselves steeped in blessings and sweetness. They tend to clothe themselves in soft velvety garments without hard edges or angles and their gestures flow as if moving in pure waters. Their voices are softly musical and transparent, with diffuse focus, wafting between heaven and earth on a cloud of feathers. Some may even seem to hover before their audience. They may feel that nothing separates them from their audience as they also softly merge with the lives of their characters. Drawing diverse worlds together, their stories may express spiritual themes and the even sublime enjoyment of the present moment.

Exercises to Explore and Balance the Spleen and Pancreas

Dynamic transformation. Referring to the characteristics listed, create a tale in which your protagonist completely transforms your antagonist.

Earth angels. Many people today have experienced invisible helping presences that mysteriously appear on the physical plane. Sit with another person to exchange accounts of your meeting with one of these visitors. Or describe a time when you found yourself unexpectedly playing the role of angelic helper for others.

If you were an angel, what guidance would you offer to your community today? How would you bring about changes?

Create a fable. Make up a story about an angel who is adjusting to the human realm.

Sugar or salt? Carry on a conversation with your pancreas about sweetness, until you feel a wild need for more down-to-earth salty talk. Or speak with such salty realism that you feel a compelling longing for genuine sweetness.

Bringing on new blood. The spleen is a gateway to fresh blood and the vehicle for each individual's unique identity. We each have a chance to bring new blood into tired and congested situations. Draw, dance, or describe in words a destructive situation at work or in your more personal life. Now introduce a story character that gently clears and refreshes the scene, perhaps leaving a mood of majestic purity and the scent of jasmine or cypress.

List how the following could be made more available in your community: organic fruits and vegetables, aromatherapy, natural medicaments, organic fibers, solar energy, and sustainable housing.

Blind trust. Lead another person whose eyes are closed gently by the hand through a garden or a house. Then reverse roles. In a larger group, keep passing the hand in your care graciously to other guardians. Then write an autobiographical tale about a time when you felt mysteriously uplifted, protected, and guided.

A protected listening space. Find a protected place in nature, or create a soft, safe story space indoors to which you can invite another, whether child or adult. Then offer that person a gentle, happy story.

Dancing polarities. Dance the expansive winged freshness of the spleen and pancreas. Then express the propelling energies of the stomach, so energetically sensitive to every intricate movement of which the body is capable. Breathe with your whole body as you dance between these polarities, giving the precise and sometimes wildly hyperactive energy of the stomach a soft ethereal dancing partner.

Expanding Spleen and Pancreas Awareness
Through Dance, Music, and Yoga

Dance

Breathe freely while standing with your arms outstretched. Waft them up over your head and then down again. Feel the pleasure of folding imaginary wings softly behind and in front of your torso. Loosen your fingers, toes, and lips, keeping your knees softly bent as you move. Fly gently, moving and turning freely, with your arms fully outstretched as if they are vast wings.

Music

Mendelssohn, The Dance of the Fairies from *A Midsummer Night's Dream*
Satie, *Gymnopédies*
Claude Debussey, *Prélude à L'Après-midi d'un Faune*
Aaron Copeland, "Simple Gifts" from *Old American Songs*

Yoga asanas (Sanskrit names in italics)

Seated Leg-Stretching Butterfly *(Purna Titali)*
Standing Leg-Stretching Poses *(Dandayamana-Bibhaktapada-Paschimottanasana)*
Garland *(Malasana)*

9

Entertainer: The Bladder

The drama of urination is fascinating to young and old. A storyteller who has achieved world fame in his adult years, began his career very early as he stood on stage for the first time to recite a nursery rhyme. When the curtain rose, he was awed to discover himself standing in a blaze of light with many eyes gazing at him, and a wet stream flowing down his leg and across the stage.

For everyone, the warm and dramatic surprise of outgoing urine is only the start in experiencing its splashy detoxifying role. We may take urine for granted, or debase it with our attitudes and words. Yet, as with all bodily functions, it is delightful to take a more accepting and enlightened view.

Westerners are usually surprised to discover that the bladder meridian runs from head to toe in the human body. Traditional Chinese medicine physicians have claimed over many centuries that this energy line originates on the inside of each eye, flowing upward over the crown of the head in two parallel channels, to dive down either side of the spine to the knees. From there it descends to encircle the outer anklebones, and skims along the bony outer edge of each foot to the tip of the littlest toes.

An easy way to stimulate this lengthy energetic pattern is to place one foot a few inches in front of the other. Then lean forward until you are supporting yourself with both hands on the floor in front of you. As you shift your weight farther forward onto your hands, lift one leg behind you. Straighten your back as you press down with your forward foot. Your littlest toe may tingle, and you will soon sense energy coursing upward from between your eyebrows, spilling over

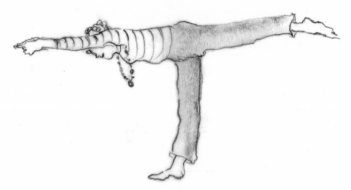

Bladder Exercise

the crown of your head and down either side of your spine. As new energy bursts into your face, you may even feel as though you are wearing a dramatic and intriguing mask and long to stand before an audience, or at least the nearest mirror. Now do the same exercise with your other foot in the forward position.

The word "bladder" comes from the Anglo-Saxon *blaedre,* meaning a flexible sac or receptacle. Like every digestive and cathartic process in the body, the work of the bladder has its own pace and rhythm. Neatly stowed in the lower front of the pelvic cavity, it provides satellite intelligence, as all our organs do, to guide the brain. With its lively outgoing sense of direction, it releases the kidneys from their inward distilling processes. As the bladder holds and regulates the flow of urine, stretching as it fills, it can accumulate as much as a quart. When it is time to urinate, a fountain spouts on its own schedule four to six times a day on average, alternating the contraction and relaxation of its muscles and nerve impulses. A fine tube at the bottom of the bladder, called the urethra, sends forth between one and two quarts a day of urine to the outer world. After a bout of urination, the bladder easily contracts again.

REDISCOVERING OLD MEDICINE

I was astonished when I first heard about the medical applications of urine. The brother of a friend of mine healed from years of painful acne in three weeks by drinking his urine and using it for massage and in his bathwater. Martha Christy claims in her book *Urine Therapy: Your Own Perfect Medicine* that taking a few drops of morning urine in a glass of water on a regular basis can cure a host of diseases, ranging from the common cold to cancer, arthritis, and AIDS.

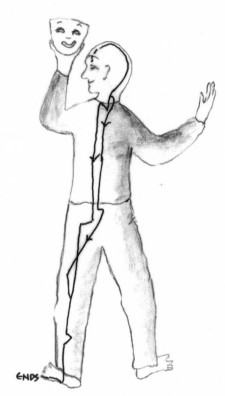

The Bladder Meridian

Medical research throughout the world indicates that urine is sterile and nontoxic. Everyone has a steady supply that contains compounds very specific to us. Urine can show the first signs of pregnancy, and has the unique quality with which animals mark their territories. Around the world, many people have learned to use their own urine externally and internally to survive injury and to enhance their life forces. This cost-free medical practice is described in one of the oldest surviving documents of Egyptian history and is being studied as an alternative medical resource. Bedouins use urine freely to treat burns, wounds, and rashes. The Aztec Indians also used urine to heal wounds. Various other cultures recommend drinking one's own urine to increase fertility and stimulate sexuality. It is also used to break down blood clots, as a sleep aid, and to cure fungal infections, fever, diabetes, cancer, and, of course, bladder problems. Ancient Chinese medical texts record specific ways to use urine and even describe how it can be purified into a powdered crystal to assuage any squeamishness on the part of the patient. In India, yogis sometimes drink urine, a practice called *shivambu*. Some indigenous Americans encountered in 1806 by Lewis and Clark's expedition to Oregon had the custom of "bathing themselves all over with urine every morning," according to Captain Meriwether Lewis. Many a sailor without a freshwater source, like recent NASA explorers, drank their own urine. Wrote one of Ferdinand Magellan's crewmen in 1519, "It was surprisingly not unsavory, having no worse a taste than a flagon of rancid port."

PERFORMANCE AS PURIFICATION

Every day the bladder performs its own intimate suspenseful drama within you. All our organs comprise a background theater for this discharging energy. The backbone acts as a lightning rod for the emotional awareness it can release throughout the body. The bladder energy pattern connects with the creativity of small intestine, the depth of the kidneys, and the intimate enticement of sexuality, supporting much of the world's best entertainment.

It is not surprising that a healthy bladder, with its flowing and often generous outbursts of urine, affects all our bodily circulations. On a hot day after a cooling drink, we may especially feel its vivid effects through the entire body. Particularly in the male body, its urges are intimately woven with sexuality, as the urethra also provides passage for semen and other seminal fluids. It brings relief and a refreshing sense of "Ahhh" and "Yes!" The collecting and releasing process of the bladder corresponds to a similar and more comprehensive dynamic process in the entire psyche. On the physical level, tubes from the kidneys, called ureters, send urine into the bladder. There, in this dusky theater, the urine waits, sometimes under pressure, producing a sense of wild anticipation.

LIGHTS, ACTION, APPLAUSE

Behind the curtains in unlit theaters, performers relish the sense of expectation as the cathartic energies of the bladder pour through them. "When I stand on stage," says a seasoned actor and film artist, "it is less performance and more surprise. I surrender to what happens on the stage and in the audience. It is beyond me." Like most performers, he feels himself stimulated by the bladder meridian to push forward from behind. "Ah, my friend," he insists, "peeing is as fundamental as breathing." With emotionally resilient backbone counterbalancing the quiet inward mood of the kidney zone, he and his theater company press forward onto stages and platforms, aiming toward full expression.

An attentive audience brings out the convivial best in bladder-strong folk. Whether stars or scenery changers, stage artists of all kinds practice and prepare their acts in hopes that everyone will enjoy and benefit from their performances as much as they do. As they respond to the vital exchange of energy, their vulnerability and urgency communicate excitement. Driven to leap up and be seen, they gather groups to marinate in the limelight along with them. They often have the knack of coaxing comedy out of serious matters, rousing joy and upliftment as they host and perform in all sorts of stage events and cabarets. Emotional and artistic, a group will often put on a show just for mutual entertainment. They get into the spirit and the show gambols along, the performers telling more and more improbable tales simply for the wild fun of it, or dressing up and acting out bits of plays and spontaneous character studies, imitating madly.

Both in their performances and communications, bladder-strong folk want and need applause. The life forces that pour into them may be so loaded with cathartic energies that they need to rouse a roar from an audience, and "blow the roof off." As the surging tide of ovations rolls back to them, helping them to feel restored and balanced, the stage can take on the energy of a revival tent. A large theater or circus tent can bring about an intimate transfer of feelings and joyous renewal. Carnegie Hall in New York City and countless stages, sports arenas, cinemas, coliseums, and music halls have been built to illuminate the power of superb performance, and to release pent-up emotions. "Lights! Action! Excitement! Leading roles! Broadway, here I come!" The bladder part of all of us loves an audience, and a cathartic standing ovation.

Nails, hairdo, makeup, glamorous theatrical outfits donned with a feeling of mounting excitement—even reclusive introverts can sometimes enjoy dressing up and stepping out to go to the theater. A bladder-strong friend of mine goes to the theater at every opportunity and loves to host costume parties, combining an amusingly serious air of business and comical exuberance.

Every morning, Hugh Morgan Hill, better known as Brother Blue, the grandfather of American storytelling, makes an offering of bread and water to lift the world through storytelling. His signature story is about the transfiguration of a humble grub into the winged beauty and freedom of a butterfly. His wife, Ruth, often helps Blue to paint bright butterflies on his forehead, the palms of his hands, and the soles of his feet. For many years in Cambridge, Massachusetts, they have made everyone welcome at their famous Tuesday story evenings. Blue also invites others to join him in the limelight on stage and radio and on his weekly television programs. Any street corner or curbside can become his stage, whether he is telling a story for a depressed student, a cat, a tree, or a harried housewife. I have seen a bag lady, a famous professor, and a pregnant mother look at one another in loving wonder as he captures the essence of each one by weaving them into a story. Brother Blue is famous for leaping barefooted onto a rickety stool or tabletop to bless his audience with a tale. Sometimes Ruth has to restrain him during other people's performances. "Don't do it!" she whispers with dignity, as he poises to leap forward onto the stage to praise others, whether professors, politicians, or performers, and to encourage applause.

Ashley Ramsden also feels a natural urge to be up and "out there." He explains, "When I walk on stage in an empty theater, I think, this is my home. I revel here! We stage folk imagine the event, the pathos of the moment, the stillness, the uproarious laughter. Even rehearsing in the living room, I sense myself on a big stage. My imagination goes wild when I am practicing in an empty theater alone, anticipating the seats full, and the buzz of the audience. I even delight in hurling myself out there when I have nothing to say. The greatest clowns have the capacity to just be there, looking at the audience and enjoying being looked at. The experience of just 'being here now' is entertainment, too." Yet Ashley warns the students who attend his School of Storytelling: "No matter how much you enjoy the limelight, storytelling is a social art. The stories and listeners you are there to serve demand a great deal of artistic and moral responsibility."

Communal catharsis is also experienced through major sports events, such as the Rose Bowl, and in the alternation of horrifying news events and playful advertising. As eager audiences come to play their part, they enhance the detoxification process. In ancient Greece, the whole population of a city would pack the amphitheater for several days' journey through the depths of tragedy and the relief of comedy. The wisdom of that time knew how to create catharsis for the well-being of the community. Today thousands gather in a natural outdoor amphitheater in northern Vermont on a huge curving green hillside to experience Peter Schumann's Bread and Puppet Theater, as nature, too, participates in the wholesome cathartic flow of the event.

In the theater of their lives, bladder folk like a good time. With a desire to please, they are destined to entertain others, even when they are "pissing around." Their talents emerge from hiding what may feel like emptiness on the inside. In the anticipation of outbursts of cheer and applause, as they prepare and practice their chosen act, they develop their keen eye for life. They may clown, standing before emptiness, picking up contradictions and absurdities, causing you perhaps to laugh until you "pee your pants." A sense of emptying and relief is followed by renewal, as a higher and subtler bladder process bubbles up and outward in the whole body and psyche of both performer and audience.

THE BACKBONE IS A LADDER TO SUCCESS

The energies of the bladder that strengthen the backbone also produce a natural drive for success, and for others to succeed. When bladder personalities are not out there performing themselves, they flourish as impresarios who organize and promote others. They facilitate the flow of events with gracious introductions and highlights of delightful commentary, and are thrilled when people enjoy an evening's entertainment. They thrive by creating a genial space for others to come forward and do whatever suits them best. As talk show hosts and hostesses, they provide an open platform for people to express themselves. They can also be public relations professionals, aiming toward product success. As sales managers, they produce images for success. Perhaps lacking scruples and depth, they can be effective "spin doctors" who set up people for success in business, politics, and other public arenas. They coach sports as performance. They have a pleasant knack for setting up courses and trainings, throwing generous parties, and creating events that celebrate others' achievements before an approving audience.

THEATER ARTS IN EVERY COMMUNITY

Just as everybody needs a well-functioning bladder, so healthy communities require at least one well-managed theater. Children as well as adults need "theatrical" experiences. In early childhood, as they gain control over their bladders, they develop imitative glee and demonstrate natural love for performance. Impressions they receive with their whole selves from the outer world flow just as naturally out of them again as they play. Children and adults sense when it is time to spread a blanket on the grass for a stage and have a talent show. Little children, like adults, may have a bout of stage fright, yet as the joyous longing to be seen wins out, the forward propulsion of singing, dancing, and other playacting releases them from anxiety. The happy exchange with their audience that results has little to do with ego gratification. Even when there is no immediate audience, an imaginary audience can do as well. Happy young children, as well as healthy actors and actresses, feel surrounded by a benevolent audience no matter what they do. As they busily go about creating their stage world, if no one is there for them, they will create an imaginary friend or two.

Whether working from a script or improvising, bladder-strong personalities often aim to transform injustice and cruelties through exposing them on stage and screen and in story. As storytellers, many are akin to shamans, who sometimes enter a village on stilts, improvising as they prepare to take willing onlookers on a cathartic healing journey that sometimes raises them to commune with spirits.

PRAISE SINGING

Bladder-strong people like to sing the praises of others and to see others praised. The singing of praises in poem and story is a skill and art. Says a seasoned storyteller, "If you introduce someone well, the audience feels good, but I cringe if anyone receives too much blatant adulation." In the past, kings and queens often appointed their official praise singers. Maya Angelou played this role for Bill Clinton in 1998. Mzwakhe Mbuli honored Nelson Mandela and his story in Capetown at his inauguration ceremonies in 1994, saying:

Let me dedicate my poetic praise / To the symbol of resistance.
Let me dedicate my poetic praise / To the symbol of hope and prosperity.
Let me dedicate my poetic praise / To the fountain of wisdom and inspiration.
I talk of Nelson Rolihalahla Mandela / The leader that stood the test of time,
Like gold and diamond / In order to be refined.
You have gone through the fires of time, Comrade Mandela. / You are like an oak tree.
You have survived all kinds of weather.

Mary Sue Siegel, a Dutch American storyteller, learned of an African custom that harnesses the power of praise in difficult circumstances. If anyone in the tribe has behaved badly, the others form a circle, place the person in the center, and speak about this person's positive qualities and achievements. No mention is made of the wrong done. Afterward, the offender simply goes on with life, steeped in praise. A teacher who witnessed this in action in Africa was so inspired by the method that she returned to her school in Holland and introduced it to the children she taught. It soon caught on. A new principal who saw a child hit another child strode across the playground. He was about to admonish the offender when his classmates quickly formed a circle to protect the boy. Then, as they had learned, they began to praise him. The principal was completely disarmed that day—it was his turn to learn.

BUILDING A SCAFFOLD OF STORIES

Abraham Lincoln once wrote, "A good story is medicine to my bones." Skeletal formations firmly give us the ability to find and to hold our own ground, and to grow. Chinese medicine has known for centuries that the energies of the bladder affect the health of our bones. Much of the immune system is cradled within them. Like the tale of young King Arthur lifting his sword out of a stone, the old English tale "Jack and the Beanstalk" fortifies the backbones of growing children. Jack sees an astonishing beanstalk in his own back garden and climbs up into an unknown land. At the top, he discovers himself in the castle of a murderous giant who has slain his father and stolen his riches. Each time he ascends to the castle, he outwits the giant and, eventually, is able to leap with the goods down the beanstalk to create a new life for his mother and himself. The beanstalk is a picture of the growing backbone and skeletal strength that encloses the cellular origin of the interior immune system.

FINDING THE TRUE SELF BEHIND THE MASK

The process of growing into oneself can be challenging for those who embody the energies of the bladder. They may have trouble differentiating life on stage from the nitty-gritty of offstage life. Behind their charm, outward success, playfulness, and business, they may feel quiet desperation and confusion. I taught "professional children" for several years in New York City. Some of my teenage students had been dancing, singing, and acting on stage and screen since they were very young. I saw for myself the challenges children face who depend from an early age on a grand audience. One of my students, who had received an Emmy award for his acting in a television program, even had the school administrators confused. He managed to buy the privilege of wearing a graduation robe to go through the motions of graduating with his class. Like the emperor who wore no clothes, he pretended successfully that he had completed the two years of work he owed to his teachers.

"Be yourself" is easy to say. "Which self?" bladder-strong folk may ask. "Always being someone else gives me confidence." When a merchant asked the Mulla Nasrudin, the famed Middle Eastern comic hero, if he could identify himself, Nasrudin was bewildered. He nervously began to extricate an amazing amount of stuff from his pockets. Finally, after much anxiety, he pulled out a small mirror, looked into it, and with much relief said, "Yes, that's me."

Show business personalities can be in danger of both finding and losing themselves in the excitement and fascination of the silvery surface of gloss, glamour, and adulation. Unbalanced, bladder energies may produce empty superficiality, all show with no real substance behind it. Some actors discover different parts of themselves in the roles they play, yet are haunted by their lack of self-knowledge. They may ask, "Who among these many characters am I really?" Part of some actors' energy may arise from a desperate feeling of not knowing themselves and yet longing for approval. They find relief and self-approval only in getting out again before a crowd.

Ovid told the sad myth of Narcissus in Book 3 of his *Metamorphosis*. It portrays a beautiful boy who could not feel for others, so absorbed was he with his own appearance. A great soothsayer had warned Narcissus that he was one who was never to be loved. Indeed, gazing into a pool of water at his reflection, he fell into his own image and drowned.

A famous Japanese myth portrays the theme of narcissism in a more positive light. It tells of a time when the Sun goddess Amaterasu hid herself in a cave.

As a result, the sky turned black and cold, and the world was afflicted by an endless night with no moon or stars to light up the sky. As long as the Sun goddess remained hidden away in the cave, there was no light or warmth. People and plants began to die. At last, other deities decided to entice her out again. They carefully constructed a mirror and hung it on a tree outside the cave. They told jokes, and the deities laughed so hard they bent over, holding their sides. Together they started to sing and dance, calling out, "Who is that delightful beautiful one?"

Inside the cave, the lonely Sun goddess heard the laughter and felt curious. She pushed the rock slightly aside and peered out. Not realizing that she was looking at her own reflection in the mirror, she said, "Let me meet this beautiful being."

A strong god waiting on the other side caught hold of the rock and pulled it completely away, until all of Amaterasu's light poured out again into the darkened world. As soon as Amaterasu was out of the cave, the other gods and goddesses embraced and held onto her firmly. "Please, stay with us," they begged. And she did.

Performing artists, though they may have a tendency to narcissism, learn to accept and serve their own rich inner integrity by focusing their energy on the inner truth of characters they portray on stage and screen. They risk losing themselves by being absorbed into a character and, as a result, neglecting themselves as they forget the integrity of their own personalities. A Celtic legend describes the ability to grow beyond appearances into deep inner truth and self-acceptance.

∾⋆∾⋆∾⋆∾

When the Mask Slips Away

Tradition maintains that if you look into a pool at midnight on Beltain eve in early May in Ireland, you will see the face of the one you are destined to love. Long ago, the liveliest of the Beltain celebrations was held at the palace of the fairy king. Along with many others, Sheronin climbed the hill at midnight to gaze into the palace lake below the fairy king's palace. There he saw a face so beautiful that it nearly broke his heart. It was the face of the daughter of the king, who was everyone's delight and heart's desire. Yet how was Sheronin to win her? All the most handsome heroes in the land courted her. Although Sheronin was kind, he was not handsome, nor was he particularly brave. He preferred to make people laugh.

After a time, he remembered the wise woman who lived nearby and went to visit her. "Good lady," he asked, "can you make me handsome?"

"Yes," she said. "I can make a mask that will fit you perfectly. With it you will take on the looks and demeanor of the handsomest hero, if that is what you *really* want. But I warn you that once you have taken on this mask, you will not be able to take it off again."

In his desperation, Sheronin agreed. When the mask was completed, Sheronin put it on. With a flourish of trumpets, he was introduced to the court. But to his dismay, the princess looked at him and exclaimed, "Not another handsome hero! I am sick of them. They are all alike, blind with love for themselves. Besides, I have seen the face of the man I am going to marry. He is not particularly comely, but he is kind. He looks like someone who could make me laugh."

"Why, that's me!" thought Sheronin. "I need only take off my mask." But whatever he did, his mask remained stuck. At last he ran back to the wise woman and begged her to help him.

"Alas," she said, "I had the power to grant your wish, but I cannot undo it."

Poor Sheronin had to return to the castle as he was. He did his best to win the hand of the princess, serving her day by day, but being a hero was not his true nature, and he became the laughing stock of the court.

One evening, filled with sorrow, he found himself walking by the palace lake. Hot tears welled within Sheronin and trickled down inside the mask. Suddenly, he felt something shift and the mask slipped from his face and landed with a splash into the water below. Sheronin looked up and laughed with relief. As he did so, he saw someone watching him, smiling from the other side of the lake. Unbeknownst to him, the princess has been walking there, too, hoping to glimpse again the face of the man she knew she was destined to love. Neither had noticed the other at first, so unhappy were they. But now they ran to meet each other. And not long afterward, a magnificent wedding feast took place.

<hr>

"Be yourself!" can be a challenge to anyone recovering from wearing a mask. A friend who is an actress and psychotherapist collects masks from every corner of the globe. Putting on these masks helps Thea familiarize herself with the grand archetypes, including goddess, witch, and shaman. She chooses them carefully. In traditional cultures, certain masks carry messages and energies beyond those of the wearer. "Each of my masks has its own lineage," she says. "They take me into experiences on the borders between the known and the unknown. They help me to dance and sing much more freely than I do in my ordinary life. When the masks are back hanging on the wall, I sometimes collapse for a while to recover from the intense awareness they inspire in my body and soul."

Tomie di Paola popularized an old French story in his children's book *The Clown of God*. It is the story of a talented boy who joins a troupe of traveling players and becomes famous for his juggling and clown masks. When he strikes out on his own as a professional juggler, he achieves even greater fame. The story begins here when he has grown old and is failing.

<hr>

The Juggler of Notre Dame

One day a crowd jeers and throws fruit at him. Tired and weary, he washes off his clown makeup and folds up his costume for the last time. It is a cold winter's night, and having nowhere to stay, he seeks refuge in a church. There he falls asleep. When he wakes, the church is blazing with light and filled with people who are bringing gifts to lay before the statue of Mary with baby Jesus in her arms. When after a time, the church is empty again, the old juggler approaches the statue, feeling ashamed that he has no gift to offer. When he looks closely, he is dismayed at the gravity of the Child's expression. Suddenly, he has an idea. He rolls out his old carpet, dons his costume, and begins to perform for the holy Mother and Child.

At that moment, one of the monks enters the church to discover the juggler, completely absorbed in his performance. The poor monk is horrified at what he sees and too quickly judges the old man. He hurries out to seek his superior. Meanwhile, the colorful balls fly higher and higher into the air as the old clown shares his gift with his whole being. At last, the heart of the old juggler gently bursts, and he falls to the ground with love. Shortly afterward, when the worried monks stream into the church, they are amazed to find him dead, and the Mother and Child smiling, a golden ball in the Child's hands.

⋅⋙⋆⋘⋅

TRANSFORMATIONAL STORYTELLING

Bladder Affirmation

I am a clear mirror.

Basic Bladder Story Dynamic

Self-display supports success for all.

Bladder Protagonists and Antagonists

Bladder protagonists (characters who support bladder health) motivate and promote. They manifest admired human qualities through excellent high-spirited events. They are cheerfully candid entertainers deserving of praise and applause, arousing delight, and even extraordinary bliss.

Bladder antagonists (characters who express bladder dysfunction) appear anxious and superficial. Hyperactive and dilettantish, they schedule an endless stream of stage events and grow overwhelmed, deceitful, and careless.

Basic Story Elements

Myths and stories often resonate with specific internal processes. This reliable pattern invokes well-being and resilience in every cell of your body:

Setting Out: The protagonist sets out in quest of greater love, strength, justice, wisdom, and happiness.

Trouble: One or more obstacles and/or antagonists interfere with the journey.

Help: Wise and benevolent help comes, often giving a gift.

Positive Ending: The protagonist fulfils the quest with joy and celebration.

SUMMONING YOUR STORYTELLER

Imagine your inner storyteller leaping barefoot onto a platform, whether a tree stump, a soapbox, or a stage. A crowd gathers immediately, responding to the excitement. An outpouring of delightful antics charms the onlookers. The storyteller's loose and flowing clothes encourage the sense of effortless exchange and upliftment. The storyteller expresses many voices, yet within their contradictions lives a dedicated personality that is positive and intact, the master of many illusions. Airy and graceful gestures complement a malleable, buoyant voice. In this generous story space, anxieties are transformed into an exciting mood of acceptance. Here a variety of characters seem to manifest before the eyes of the audience, as the storyteller expresses for them the very things holding them back from living more freely.

Exercises to Explore and Balance the Bladder

Who is that delightful one? Although we are all attached to our own usual introverted or extroverted moods and way of speaking, the bladder's energies move us to an extroverted outpouring of showmanship. Name a wonderful quality you would like to have more of in your life, such as playfulness or wonder. Now imagine yourself wearing a mask that displays that quality. Children easily perform before an imaginary audience. Imagine yourself giving an exciting performance to grand applause. Now go ahead and invite an audience, even if the audience you choose to have is only your cat. If it is evening or dark, place candles for your footlights.

Disappearing and being there. Put yourself down a "rabbit hole" and feel yourself disappearing for a time. Then walk through a looking glass and become as marvelously visible to the whole world as possible.

Creating a stage, expecting applause. Create a simple stage. Throw a cloth down on the lawn or in your living room. Let it be a stage and step onto it.

What kind of audience would you like to summon for your performance? Imagine grand applause before you begin. Be sure that you bow and express your thanks for the spectators' willing participation and the excitement of having this attention.

Singing praises. "Praise is simply drawing back the curtains," wrote the great poet Rumi. On special occasions, storytellers practice praise singing. Interview another person about the important facts of his or her life, including attitudes, beliefs, and accomplishments large and small. Ask: "Who nurtured you? When did you begin to experience your own path? What obstacles have you overcome? Describe some of your most triumphant moments." Then compose a rhythmic eulogy extolling the spirit, the virtues, and the many accomplishments of this person. Create an occasion to deliver this oration, perhaps at a birthday party or other special time. Imagine you are standing at the top of a waterfall to practice singing these praises. Standing on a stool or table to deliver your praise song will give the feeling of being on stage, if a stage is not available.

Depression results from the refusal to praise. Write about an important moment in your life as story song. Then stand on a chair or table and deliver your praise song to the world.

The wandering mask-maker. Make up a story about a wandering mask-maker who can provide exactly the mask that is needed. Continue the story by telling about someone who is changed by a mask into which, for better or for worse, he or she grows into.

The shaman behind the mask. Imagine that you are a village shaman whose antics bring catharsis to a whole tribe. Make up a story about that inspired healer.

Sharing the limelight. Scene 1. Designate half of a group as audience and half as performers. The performers try anything to catch the attention of the audience.

Scene 2. Do what you can to graciously bring someone else into the limelight.

Scene 3. Interview someone and then introduce that person to the group, praising his or her accomplishments and virtues.

EXPANDING BLADDER AWARENESS THROUGH DANCE, MUSIC, AND YOGA

Dance

Raise one leg up behind you and hold it there for a few moments, lifting your face as you bend forward. Press both arms against your standing leg, or against the floor. Now reverse legs. Then imagine that you are wearing an exciting mask and dance forward as if to meet a huge audience. Or imagine that you are dancing with a mirror and discover what your body does as you change your expressions to express different moods, such as wonder, grief, joy, amusement, and surprise.

Music

Riccardo Drigo, *Harlequinade*
Bernstein, *West Side Story* Dance at the Gym
Weber, *Phantom of the Opera* orchestrated
Piovani, *La Vita è Bella*
Jarre, *Witness* Building the Barn

Yoga asanas (Sanskrit names in italics)

Airplane *(Tadasana)*
Striding Forward Bend *(Uttanasana)*
Warrior 3 *(Virabhadrasana)*
Lunge *(Ashwa Sanchalasana)*
One Leg Balancing Forward Bend *(Tuladandasana)*
Standing Bow *(Dandayamana-Dhanurasana)*

10

Quiet Sage: The Kidneys

Human kidneys are bean-shaped twins, each about as big as the palm of your hand. Watery seeds saturated with cosmic wisdom, like all seeds, each holds and protects profound secrets of life. By a gentle process in the deep reservoir of the body, the kidneys work together to balance minerals and to help regulate the waters in all of our cells. Alchemists of our daily urine, in a huge water exchange, they absorb ten liters to every one liter sent down to the bladder for excretion.

Whether absorbing or excreting, the kidneys are uniquely sensitive organs. Like every organ, they serve our whole being. Deep within the torso, well protected between backbone and ribs, they radiate energy upward to the heart and lungs. Beyond our modern concept of two sleek biological organs, in their larger invisible function, through the sway of our blood and breathing, they regulate much of our subtle feeling life. "Trailing clouds of glory," they help every inhalation of breath to include the mysterious far reaches of our origins. They cause our senses to stream together as a whole and help us to listen and speak from the unifying waters of life. They also strengthen bone joints and stimulate sensitivity to the joining places between all things.

During the nine months of human gestation, embryonic kidneys resemble tiny deities in meditation, listening in boundless seas as they gradually migrate down from either side of our ears to settle firmly within us. Throughout our lives, they continue to communicate vibrant echoes of the generative seas from which we spring. On the threshold between land and water, like a gentle harpist, they tune to subtle sea swells within our bodies.

To study a kidney with a microscope is rather like peering inside a butterfly chrysalis to find the hidden power of transfiguration. The physiology of the kidneys has kept medical researchers busy over many years inventing increasingly subtle ways to observe and measure their activities. Exquisite pyramid-shaped chambers inside each kidney receive and filter blood and other liquids, salts, and toxins left over from digestive processes. These liquids gradually etherealize as they move through miles of minute delicate arterial vessels compressed within the pyramids and radiate via a distilling process into the formative energies around the body. This sets up a streaming of delicate sensations and images, and lends a quality of deep refinement to the whole body and soul.

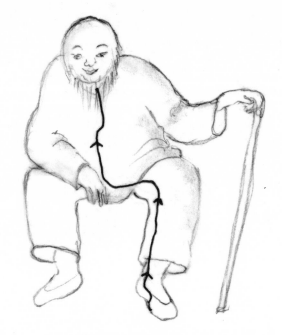

The Kidney Meridian

According to traditional Chinese medicine physicians, the journey of kidney energy begins underneath the littlest toes and emerges along the arches of the feet. It curves behind the inner anklebones and ascends along the inside of our knees to penetrate the torso near the coccyx bone at the base of the spine. There these lines connect with both kidney and bladder, before flowing upward over the abdomen and chest.

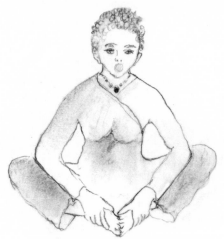

Kidney Exercise

A branch ascends through the liver and diaphragm and enters the lungs, branching along the throat and emptying into the delta at the root of the tongue. Another branch joins the heart from the lung and connects with the meridian flow of the heart protector, the pericardium.

EXPERIENCING KIDNEY ENERGY

To feel the quiet strength of the kidneys deep within you, lie on your back, let your knees fall apart, and press the soles of your feet together. Or press the soles of your feet together as you sit upright. Try to match all the toes of one foot with the toes of the opposite foot. In this natural meditative position, contract your knees inward and at the same time open them outward. Straighten your spine. Following this method, I have seen deep inward concentration surprise even the most skeptical extroverts.

The kidneys extract and liberate. Both of these functions are important for people in whose personality kidney energy predominates. The kidneys tend to pare life quickly down to essentials. Paradoxically, at the same time they give us an expansive sense of freedom to grow and to unfold new capacities. In Western esoteric tradition, the kidneys are connected with the goddess Venus, often visualized rising from the depths of the sea, her wise and beautiful body as buoyant as Noah's ark. Amidst vast destructive forces, the kidneys, like Venus and Noah, preserve and guard the most sacred powers of regeneration. Those who express the kidney realm in their personalities especially value depth and integrity. From their silence springs sensitive and deep listening that calms physical aggression.

The kidney tribe, which is scattered throughout all human cultures, tends to be profound, pithy, and poised. Its people often speak their truth in few words. The more they listen, the more they are able to find words and wisdom that generate a unified outlook. Mary Oliver's poetry portrays this mood. She asks in "Leaf and Cloud":

Would it be better to sit in silence,
To think everything,
To feel everything, to say nothing.

Like a motionless and concentrated seed holds the secrets of life, kidney personalities shun disturbances and small talk. Their ambition is often to create peace, insight, and enlightenment for all. By their very presence, they sublimate, transmute, and redeem. After listening to several long and rambling stories, a wise kidney-tuned student said, "Well, here's *my* story." After a pause she spoke only these words: "Bring the Lamp into the room."

SILENT LISTENERS

People who live absorbed in such introverted secrets tend to wonder at noisier, more casual lifestyles. Their protective peaceful aura quiets and calms others. From their inwardness, delicate light emanates, reminiscent of starlight. Bathed in this cosmic glow, they often see what others do not, as their inner light radiates into all their senses, expanding and opening them like gentle flowers. It is not surprising that these people avoid superficial pleasures, walk out of even the finest restaurants if they are noisy, and only reluctantly turn on electronic entertainments. They tend to retreat into corners in a mood of deep quietness. The mute mysteries of the seed glimmer in their eyes and presence. They can seem to be there, and to not be there at the same time, like the hero of "The Twelve Dancing Princesses," who follows the princesses secretly into their watery night world. They listen deeply for rich universal tones sounding within and around them. Seekers of transcendental truth, insincerity and superficiality repel them.

Kidney-strong folk cherish wise jokes, such as these:

A musician banished to Siberia at last found an old battered violoncello with only one string. Hearing him play the same note on that one string steadily for hours, his wife grew exasperated. She shouted, "Husband, can't you play a melody?" He replied calmly, "Everyone has been looking for the right note, dearest. I have found it."

A sixty-year-old man met a wizard and was granted one wish. After some thought, he said, "I would like my wife to be thirty years younger." Suddenly, he discovered that he had become ninety years old.

The Waters of Truth

When I invite groups to imagine a storyteller who embodies the concentrated inwardness of the kidneys, I enjoy how similar these imaginary storytellers often are. A woman pictured a child-like old man who was dressed in soft mosses and bark. His "storytelling" was a quiet communing with water, birds, and trees as birds and nature spirits nested in his hair and ears. He carried a harp and flute from which pure tones flowed. As she connected with the deep waters of truth concentrated within her, another course participant discovered a similarly intriguing inhabitant of the kidney realm: "To be near Babushka felt tremendously rich. Looking into her eyes was like falling into a deep pond, where all answers and questions peacefully unite."

Much great literature is written because the author wants to share unusual subtle experiences that arise from the radiant strength of the kidneys. Through inspired, attentive, deep listening, fabulous eloquence can unexpectedly emerge from this deep energy center, even from children. Like William Blake, the throng who inhabit this realm tend to find "a world in a grain of sand, eternity in an hour," and the power to transform hell into heaven through belief in human potential.

Their words whirr, set between the fire of thought and the water of feeling. Their condensed thoughts and feelings strive inward toward unity, and outward beyond space and time toward infinite horizons. Through an inward process of sensing deep underlying causes, they understand using more than logic and learning. The depth of their contemplative awareness can be startling and disconcerting to others. Their silence can grow huge wings of inspiration.

The profound seeker within us recognizes the need for wholeness and senses "learning edges," rejoicing at possibilities and new strengths forming. This seeker naturally wants to acknowledge the higher consciousness within each person, and to distill and release toxic shadows. As poets and sages, kidney folk often lead singularly puzzling and inspiring lives, longing to share the depth of their sensitivities. Near the end of his career, attuned more to ethereal realities than to solid matter, Shakespeare wrote *The Tempest,* a play crammed with watery and aerial kidney themes.

Before his twentieth birthday, the English poet John Keats trained as a physician. He learned the parts of the body—nerves, bones, sinews, muscles—by dissecting cadavers provided by body snatchers who had robbed churchyards of their corpses. While he walked the wards and assisted during operations, like many deep souls, he woke from illness and death to restore his vitality eventually in a lush and passionate flow of poetic utterance.

The profound folk who inhabit the kidney zone seek beauty for relief from their hypersensitivity, and often reveal a hidden streak of playfulness. The Sufi poet Rumi wrote:

> *When I die, lay out*
> *my body like a corpse.*
> *You may want to kiss my lips*
> *just beginning to decay.*
> *Don't be surprised*
> *if I open my eyes.*

Within everyone live deep waters that may arise unexpectedly with a spray of sparkling understanding. Rumi's poem expresses ironic mischief. It opens a window in the soul to let in fresh air. The zany spirit that jokes in the midst of despair creates a surprising game of peekaboo to joggle fixations. Fear turns into wild ingenuity.

When we feel as if we are falling apart, the kidneys quietly preserve the will to live. One day as a young teacher, I closed the door on an uproarious class of eight-year-olds, and leaned my head against the wall in the corridor outside the classroom. Though my confidence had gone out like a light, my kidneys were nevertheless shining into my deeper self without my conscious awareness, searching for survival tactics. Next moment, as I reopened the door to the classroom, a very uplifting and hearty alter ego made herself known. Out of the genetic seed force stored within me, Mrs. MacIver manifested grandly from within me, an outspoken, feisty grandmother who had raised "seventeen children of her own" back in Ireland. "What's going on here?" she shouted in a full-blown Irish lilt. "Your teacher is out in the hall looking quite pale." My classroom full of children took to Mrs. MacIver at once, and with grateful schizoid glee, so did I.

Forging the Inner Chalice

As healthy kidney energy rises and supports survival, whether through playful ingenuity or deep quiet listening, kidney strength draws the whole life force inward and removes blocks to internal integrity. As it supports strong and supple joints, on the soul level it creates sensitivity to subtle connections. Kidney-strong folk tend to trust their own senses and see through superficialities and illusion as they listen to the heart of life and inmost kernels of meaning.

King Janaka

Once there lived a king who was also a teacher, and regarded by many as a saint. One day a student came to the palace where he was living, hoping to learn from him. The king welcomed him and bade him sit at the royal table. That night there was feasting and dancing and royal entertainment, to which the king acted as a gracious host. The student was puzzled. How could the king have such a rich reputation as a holy man? The entertainment continued night after night, so much so that the student soon forgot why he had come and began to believe that this was the way to live.

Then one day the king took him aside, saying," Dear, sir, have you seen this place?"

"Why, yes," answered the young man.

"I should like to show it to you," the king went on, and he handed the student a brimming cup of liquid.

"Follow me," said the king, "and be careful not to spill a drop."

They proceeded through the temporal delights of the palace, down to the pleasure gardens and the dancing halls. The student, eager not to spill a drop of the liquid, could not allow anything to distract him.

When they returned to the place from which they had started, the king asked, "Well, what did you think of the palace?"

"I'm sorry, my lord. To tell the truth, I did not see any of it, I was so busy carrying the bowl."

"Do not apologize" was the king's reply. "This is how I live in the palace of earthly desire. The only way I can live in it is by holding the stillness that you have just discovered."

JOY RISES FROM ABYSMAL CIRCUMSTANCES

A therapist and father of three challenging teenage sons quietly and thoughtfully attended a storytelling as a healing story group, and astonished us during the final presentations when he leapt up, donned a rakish hat, and became a storyteller from an imaginary country on the edge of the world. His persona announced in a mysterious thick accent: "I vant to tell you a story." The story was about a man who experienced depths that shook his whole soul and the storyteller related it with the same thick accent throughout.

Gamuchi and the Abyss

In our country, Kalamar, lived a man named Gamuchi. Some thought he was crazy, but he was not so crazy that he could not be put to work. So we gave him the job of collecting and discarding the garbage. But this was not ordinary garbage. In our country, when we want to discard our hatred, envy, bitterness, stupidity, and many other such things, we want to put this as far away as we can. And so Gamuchi was given the job of removing this waste from Kalamar.

The abyss at the edge of Kalamar was the only place where these burdens could be discarded so that they would not pose any threat. Gamuchi would gather a load, stand right at the edge of the steep cliff, and throw it over the edge. He would not look but he was terrified. He knew there was no bottom to this hole, and it seemed to him that big, ugly monsters lived in the depths below. The quicker he got away from there, the better he felt.

To make his job easier, Gamuchi fed the birds every day, and he got to know birds so well that they started to land on his shoulders and keep him company as he did his work. Eventually, he thought he knew what they were singing to him, and this is what he heard:

If you want to fly you must sing.
Sing and sing until your heart learns how.

For many years, Gamuchi listened to the birds as he quietly continued his frightening work. One day as he was tossing a load of malice and arrogance over the rim of the abyss, there came a deep roar from below. But Gamuchi had no choice but to collect the trash as usual. The birds tried to cheer him up. He threw a full load over the edge and at once a crack appeared in the ground. He quickly jumped onto solid land as the chunk he was standing on tumbled into the abyss below. Right away another crack appeared, and again the ground where Gamuchi stood threatened to fall into the abyss. Again he jumped, just in time. It was eerie that there was no sound of crashing at the bottom. Gamuchi ran back to town again as fast as he could.

One day as he approached the edge of the abyss with a load of greed and self-pity, his foot slipped, and this time he fell in! As he fell, Gamuchi was filled with fear, and he started to give up hope that he would survive. Just then, a bird flew toward him and started singing. Then he heard another, and another. The birdsong filled him with joy and he began to sing, and as he did he stopped falling. Gamuchi sang as he never had before, and when he stretched out his arms he began to fly. He flew right out of the abyss.

Someone in the village noticed the strange sight in the sky and told others. When the people could no longer deny that something extraordinary was happening, they gathered around Gamuchi as he landed. As he told them his story, they were astounded.

Gamuchi became a hero in Kalamar. He started a school to teach people how to fly. He had many students, and I was one of the first to learn. One day Gamuchi went off into the forest to be with the birds. After three days, he returned and told the people of his village the birds had revealed to him what he must do. He appointed a group of helpers to collect all the burdensome waste into bags and fly with it high into the air. Eventually, it dispersed and disappeared. But before it did so, it danced wonderfully intricate and beautiful patterns. We started to dance the same patterns, and doing this filled us with joy. Some of us used the patterns in our work as artists, potters, and craftspeople. Others adapted the patterns for tunes and melodies, and made beautiful music. Even those who did not consider themselves artists began to live their lives in ways that were more profound and creative. A new peace emerged in our land.

Anyway, because of Gamuchi, my country is now a place where our people are happier, and willing to let others be who they are, no matter how different they may be. And if they become difficult to live with, a visit to the abyss puts things in perspective.

༺✿༻✿༺✿༻

As the story ended, the storyteller taught the whole group to dance to the liberation song, like liberated kidney energy that rises into heart and lungs:

If you want to fly you must sing,
Sing and sing, until finally your heart learns how to sing.

STAGNANT KIDNEY ENERGY TRANSFORMS

No one entirely escapes the abyss of Kalamar. As our souls attune to the minutely complex tasks of the kidney, we feel ourselves withdrawing into deep inward mysteries. We may feel like Ceridwen's cauldron in the Welsh tradition, which must be quietly stirred for a year and a day before the universe is renewed from the magical contents within it.

A friend of mine, an actor and professional storyteller, tells me that he lives all day and night in the damp, dissolving aspect of the kidneys. As he tries to live a normal life, he feels his whole self constantly and eerily disappearing. Everyone who knows him feels his distress. At times he experiences paralyzing and devastating isolation and loss of a sense of meaning and form. He feels stricken by the heaviest thoughts and feelings. Yet, whenever he steps on stage to perform, he emerges from his dark cocoon. He soars brilliantly out of his misery when he invites comedy and laughter to play through him and lighten the still, dark core of his being.

Scrooge, the miserly hermit in Charles Dickens' *A Christmas Carol,* also rises out of depression into brilliant activity. As the intense contraction of his hermit years releases, he gladly makes a buffoon of himself. At the beginning of Dickens' masterpiece, Scrooge is a "bah-humbug" rotting and sclerotic goblin-like old man. He has bent over his accounts for so long that all his joints ache. With an empty ghostly face, he is a wizened shell of his true self. Yet in the story he is given one last merciful chance to see the truth of his life. With the help of authentic Christmas spirit, he transfigures his miserly dysfunctional kidney contraction and experiences the luminous expansiveness of heart and lungs. With Tiny Tim's "God bless us, every one!" resounding in his ears, he completely transforms his life into one of loving care for others.

Anyone who lives strongly in the kidney zone knows this Scrooge phenomenon. Healthy kidney-strong people who see ghosts or sense them in some other way, may also liberate them. When I meet people who feel their lives have become a dry, ghostly husk, I remember Scrooge, and also the plant world. Within all of us sleep concentrated seeds of life that are awaiting favorable conditions for growth. I often encourage people in my workshops to write the saga of a seed's unfolding. An artist who was longing for her own creativity to flourish wrote:

> Once upon a time, a seed lived in the deepest part of the earth. This seed was tender and ripe, yet the weight of the earth pressed so heavily that it could scarcely breathe. Out in the farthest point of the universe, a star expanded and shone into the earth's crust. The soft seed, struggling in its sleep, was awakened. Each time the star breathed, a part of the seed was drawn upward toward the heavens. As the star breathed out, it was drawn more deeply downward to explore the Earth. In this way the plant both rooted and grew, until it burst through the earth's crust. Its leaves unfurled, and there soon appeared infinitely lovely star-flowers.

Understanding the sensitivity of kidney folk can help them to show their strengths to others. Many fairy tales and wonder tales reveal heroes and heroines who, with sensitivity beyond ordinary listening, are able to serve others. A version of "The Three Languages," a middle European tale among the many collected by the Brothers Grimm, tells of a count who sent his son away to study.

⁓✾⁓✾⁓

The Three Languages

Each time the count's son returned to his father's home, the count asked, "My boy, what have you learned?"

The boy replied, "Father, I have learned what the animals know and the birds say when they are singing."

"Is that all?" the irate father shouted.

At last the count called to his servants and ordered them to take the boy to the forest and slay him because he was a disgrace. But the servants took pity on the boy and set him on a good path to another castle. There he was sent to the dungeon to sleep for the night. The king of that place warned him of wild dogs kept in the dungeon because they had been attacking the villagers. The boy asked for some pieces of meat to feed them.

All night long, he listened to the dogs tell their story. Her heard about how the villagers had been cutting down the trees in the forest and killing the animals that lived there. The next morning, the king, amazed that the boy was still alive, listened attentively to what he had to say, and took the message to the people. Soon the villagers showed more respect for the forests and creatures, and the dogs stopped attacking them.

After a time, the good king said to the lad, "I do not have a son. Would you be my adopted son and rule my kingdom when I die?"

Well, the boy was not expecting this. A white dove landed on his shoulder, singing, "Do what your heart desires."

And so it was that the boy became a prince, and cared for the villagers and the animals and trees of the surrounding forest for the rest of his life.

⋯⋰⋱⋯

TRANSFORMATIONAL STORYTELLING
Kidney Affirmation
All life connects within me.

Basic Kidney Story Dynamic
Emptiness turns into joyous awareness.

Kidney Protagonists and Antagonists
Kidney protagonists (characters who support kidney health) are sensitive, holistic thinkers and loners who seek peace and depth. They are very observant advisors. As they learn to transform their fears, they are compassionate and gentle, sensing sacred life principles in themselves and others. Original thinkers, they expand the horizons of others with insight and understanding.

Kidney antagonists (characters who express kidney dysfunction) are self-effacing, confused, and detached from emotions and relationships. They tend to be hypersensitive and shy introverts who see themselves as left out of groups.

Basic Story Elements

Myths and stories often resonate with specific internal processes. This reliable pattern invokes well-being and resilience in every cell of your body:

Setting Out: The protagonist sets out in quest of greater love, strength, justice, wisdom, and happiness.

Trouble: One or more obstacles and/or antagonists interfere with the journey.

Help: Wise and benevolent help comes, often giving a gift.

Positive Ending: The protagonist fulfils the quest with joy and celebration.

SUMMONING YOUR STORYTELLER

Storytellers in the kidney realm invoke the silence from which everything comes, and to which it must return. They speak from a deep listening place, waiting for inspiration to unfold within them. Their eyes gaze inward toward the essential creative source of all things and their voices reverberate with this deep inwardness. They wait for words to form. Resonating with the vast creative resources stored within, they listen to what these say, often feeling their words are not so much their own as issuing from a wise prompter or guide. They stand in the presence of what they have spoken, as much as any other listener. Their gestures are minimal, spare, meaningful. Nothing is extraneous; their clothing is intentionally self-effacing.

Exercises to Explore and Balance the Kidneys

Listening to silence. Close your eyes and silently listen to your own body. Seek the deepest stillness within you. Holding on to this stillness, extend your listening to the sounds in the room where you are. Now expand your listening to what is outside the room. Listen into the stillness of a flower, a tree, an owl.

Using pastels, draw a mandala-like form with a strong, deep center. Then close your eyes. Leaving words and images behind, go into your deepest self to find a still point. Remembering this still point, open your eyes.

Describe someone you know, perhaps yourself, who has deep inwardness and sensitivity and who often seeks silence, stillness, and depth (at times with a streak of pithy humor).

Meeting the wise hermit. Find a comfortable place to sit, close your eyes, and breathe deeply and peacefully. Invite the wisdom of seeds to inspire you. Imagine a wise woman or man who lives hidden in a deep, still landscape. Look closely at this figure from head to toe. Held in the hands of this sage is a gift that has the power to transform death into life. As you return to more ordinary awareness, write in a notebook about this protagonist. Then create a story about a tired, confused, introverted wanderer who is helped by this sage.

Create an Om-ing place. Remember that the kidneys regulate and distill all the waters of your body, giving a sense of preservation and vast potential as they support your breathing and heart rhythms. They awaken insight from deep within that sheds light on negativity and darkness in your inner ecosystem. Imagine a quiet and protected space that is completely attuned to the deep inward processes of your kidneys. Organize such a meditative space in your home or office.

Seeds of transformation. The kidneys radiate sensitive quiet awareness of the inner life of trees, flowers, and all the natural world. With peaceful clarity, commune with a dormant seed. What quietly dreams within an acorn? Write the growth saga of a seed, or the transformation of a grub into a butterfly, avoiding scientific words and phrases.

Imagine you are a seed of the person you want to become. What seed force awakens, germinates, and, surrounded by fine mists and rainbows, wants to combust with fiery new will?

Biographical seed times. Growth stops at times for plants and for humans. Yet a period of silence and stillness can be amazingly fertile. Seeds eventually release the fullness of what is stored within. Recall a time of repose and silence in your own or another person's life. Write about this period of fertile resting. What emerged from that quiet stillness?

EXPANDING KIDNEY AWARENESS THROUGH DANCE, MUSIC, AND YOGA

Dance

Imagine that you have ended a dance and are sitting beside a deep rock pool; beneath this pool is an ocean of knowing. A star resonates through the center of your head down to your tailbone. Sit with the soles of your feet together and your back as erect as possible. Birthless, deathless, draw yourself together inwardly to become completely still. Enjoy this stillness, as you imagine stars and planets whirling within and around you.

Music

Bells
Arvi Pärt, *Nunc Dimittis*
Vaughan Williams, *The Lark Ascending*
Blessed silence

Yoga asanas (Sanskrit names in italics)

Bound Angle *(Baddha Konasana)*
Lotus Corpse *(Savasana)*

11

Boundary Keeper: The Skin

Our human skin is a seamless garment we wear for a lifetime. With its traceries of celestial and hairy animal lineage, it tells a long evolutionary saga. A sense for friend or foe arises quickly within it. Lovers especially experience its swift repatterning, as animal-like sensations awaken on the surface of the body in the midst of lovemaking, and, as suddenly, the skin may feel permeated with angels.

Modern medicine identifies three layers of our most extensive organ as endoderm, mesoderm, and exoderm. In the deepest, endoderm layer of the skin, blood joins with metabolism. In the mesoderm, sensitive capillaries feed muscle fibers, and mix with glandular secretions, arousing zest and the vigorous joy of movement. The outmost, exoderm layer, when looked at through a magnifying glass, resembles a multitude of stars. Just as Earth wears a sparkling skin of stars, so does our skin. We can sense that under the stars this iridescent mantle of nerve-rich skin, with its many millions of point-like nerve endings, has been imprinted from far beyond our present physical boundaries.

Cinderella receives three layers of spiritual and physical protection from her mother's love: a golden dress as warm as the shining sun, a dress as reflective and silvery as the moon, and a dress as brilliantly sparkling as the stars. Ethnic garments often mirror the shimmering cosmic realities in our visible skin, and in the usually invisible light body that surrounds and protects our physical form.

As an ingenious boundary-maker, with many guards that keep watch inside and around the body, our skin is the supple meeting place for outer and inner impressions. Its sensory nerve endings can respond with great swiftness and subtlety to pressures from the external world. The skin plays out its strategies to enhance pleasure and avoid pain; to welcome and embrace; or to flee, or fight with raw defiance. It protects us body and soul, and serves as an intricate alarm system.

In this protective sheath, much of the work of the external immune system takes place. As the vulnerable life within us continuously forms its own protective covering, even if our conscious mind is not asking for protection, all three layers of skin fulfill their role as defender of the bounds. They are often on high alert in our present world. To feel less vulnerable in body and soul, we muster physical training, protective armor, and horrifying and ingenious weaponry. The toxic stockpiles of armaments throughout the world darkly mirror our overstressed global immune response.

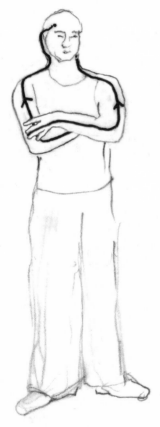

The Triple Burner Meridian

To activate the healthy flow of the skin's energy patterning, contract all your muscles for a moment and press down with your heels. To those unfamiliar with this energetic pattern, it can be astonishing to realize the intensity of the impulses and inner life generated as the skin comes alive. Roll up your sleeves and admire your forearms. Then place your hands firmly on your thighs. Breathe quickly in and out through your nose, keeping your mouth closed. Contract your belly with each exhalation. Keep this up for a few moments. In the afterglow, you will feel your skin begin to glisten with a blend of Athenian sensitivity and tough Spartan rigor.

The traditional Chinese medicine term for the meridian that is related to the skin is Triple Burner. This fiery energy system draws the body and soul together into a network of physically oriented, ardent communications that help regulate the whole body's relationship with the surrounding world. Beginning on the outer tip of the ring finger, this meridian runs upward outside the elbows and arms into the shoulders and the breastbone, and then proceeds downward to unite complex protective energies in the upper, middle, and lower body. A branch also ascends from the shoulder and circles the face, to connect with the gallbladder meridian at the outer curve of the eyebrows.

BUILDING THE EXTERIOR IMMUNE SYSTEM

A dazzling dancer who lives strongly in touch with the life of her skin claims that her skin is "an amazing sock to live inside of." She says, "I am grateful to my skin because it contains me and gives me such pleasure. It is the threshold through which I experience the world and find my true feelings about it." When she was a child, she lived with an abusive uncle; by reading fairy tales, she gradually developed immunity to his behavior, and a soul-skin as powerful as her physiological immune system. In her childhood, she especially loved the Grimms' tale "The Six Swans." In this story, the sister sewed mantles of nettles to save her brothers until her fingers bled. "I believe that we must be willing to undergo painful experiences," the dancer insists. "Through them we are able to reach truly happy endings. When I feel danger, I sometimes feel my skin expands and becomes airy and open. Then it is as if my body comes back into my skin, telling me what to do."

Though the dancer outgrew fairy tales, she continued to reach out and touch others, and makes a practice of appreciating her own skin. "Every morning I massage my whole body with my hands. Then I take long showers and baths with different scrubbers, soaps, and oils. I like to feel them on my bare skin. As a child," she muses, "I loved to see wounds healing. I was very proud of the scars on my skin, because I felt brave and alive watching the healing process." As an adult, she often dreams of swords, knives, and fencing, and is drawn to people with the ability to pierce and be pierced, and yet survive.

She is like the multitude of others who etch or pierce their skin to draw attention to their toughness and painful inner struggles, as if to say: "I am powerful. Take care to read my skin." Soon after the painful ending of her long marriage, she went to be tattooed. She chose a butterfly tattoo for her lower back caudal vertebrae and a snake for her right pelvis bone. "I screamed all through the tattooing process from the great physical pain, yet I also embraced the whole ordeal. Afterward I had beautiful emblems on my skin, permanent visible memories of all I had survived in my marriage."

Those who live predominantly under the skin's influence tend to enjoy different kinds of arduous physical challenges. Those with a strong exterior immune response quickly discern whether friend or foe is approaching across the jungle, down the street, across the dance floor. At best, they inspire in others an exhilarating sense of health and grace. Professional dancers, athletes, surfers, and musicians often start training at a very young age and are attracted to the repetition of steady practice. They enjoy the experience of gradually gaining prowess. When they are not being physically active, they look forward to extraordinary attainments and competitions.

My goddaughter Dove announced to her nonathletic parents when she was three years old that she was going to be an Olympic skater, insisting that they take her to a rink. For the next ten years, they watched her gain proficiency on the ice until, as a teenager, she announced that she would rather be a champion cellist.

Prowess in physical lovemaking and in combat often go together. The skin enjoys experiences of very physical lovemaking, whether real or imaginary. It enjoys hair-raising feats of physical prowess, riding bucking broncos, escapes from tight places, and fabulous wrestling matches. When fully aroused, like a porcupine throwing its quills in extreme self-defense, it thrills to the power of weaponry, often leaving a wake of destruction.

The transformation of raw aggression into devoted and loving closeness shines in many stories, such as this Arabian tale.

⚜⚜⚜⚜

Love in a Garden

Long ago there lived a lovely pearl of a girl who every day went to a beautiful, aromatic garden. As winds danced around her, she sang and scattered crumbs to feed the doves that visited the garden. One day, as a youth was hunting nearby with his hawk, a frightened dove took refuge in her garden, but before it could reach the protection of the trees, the hawk swooped and killed it. The girl cried as she picked up the broken bird. The hunter, following the flight of his hawk, suddenly burst into the garden. His heart turned to fire when he saw her beauty.

"Just go away!" was her response.

The young man thought, "I will bring her more doves to make up for the one that died!" He gathered his nets and his traps and for days he hunted. He captured many doves and brought them to her in a cage, but she was furious.

"These are the same doves that visited me every day and ate my crumbs. Let them go!"

He released the doves, but he could not eat nor sleep. He stopped hawking and hunting, and sat at home dreaming only of his beloved. At last he took his nets and traps, went into the hills, and caught a rare bird. Then he ran to the garden and set the cage at her feet. "For a rare girl," he said.

She looked down. The poor bird lay dead in the cage. The young man became a pearl diver. After many months, he had filled a bag with pearls. He returned to the garden and placed the pearls at the girl's feet. "Pearls for a pearl," he said.

"I don't need pearls! They belong to the sea," said she.

The hunter set sail for a distant land, prospected and dug in the ground until he had filled a chest with gold. He returned to the garden and fell on his knees before her. "Please take this gold and let me be your friend," he begged.

"What will I do with gold you stole from the earth?" was her reply.

The young hunter was in total despair. Finally, he went to a wise woman who lived on a nearby mountain. "I love her. I can't live without her. I have offered her birds and pearls and gold."

The old woman laughed. "Look in the forest and in the meadow. What do the creatures give to one another?" She offered him a small flute.

He didn't understand. As he made his way through the forest, he saw two gazelles walking side by side, softly brushing against each other. "Oh, if only I had my bow and arrow!" he thought. He heard a soft sound above him. He looked up and there sat two doves on a branch. They were rubbing their bills together and cooing gently to each other. "Oh, if only I had a stone!" he thought. As he watched, he started to envy them. He remembered his beloved and her anger. He asked himself, "How did this dove earn love? How did the gazelle earn love? What is their secret?"

He practiced on his flute for many days, and then one day he saddled his horse and galloped to the garden. "What have you brought me now?" asked the young woman sadly.

Without a word, he sat down in front of her, pulled his flute from his vest, and began to play. Out poured the longing and sweetness and pain and joy that had been locked in his heart. Softly, the music twirled up through the trees.

Soon the two of them were strolling side by side through the flowers. Beneath the shimmering leaves, they talked of everything except hunting and hawking and looking for gold.

After a time, the hunter returned to the old woman. He was soft and alight with love. She took one look at him and smiled. "Now you know what the gazelle knows and what the dove knows," she said.

⁂

Boosting Immune Response and Morality

Every response can be transformed through effort. The skin's active immune response can support miracles of strength and a moral stance that is open and caring, not hostile, and that defends the needs of others as much as one's own. The warrior hero and heroine become vigorous partners, caring about the whole shining web of life.

A twelve-hundred-year-old prophecy tells of the coming of Shambhala warriors at a time when all life on Earth is in danger because great barbarian powers have arisen. These powers spend their wealth in preparations to annihilate one another. They have in common weapons and technologies of unfathomable destructive power. In this era, the kingdom of Shambhala must arise in the hearts and minds of chosen warriors. They wear no uniforms or insignia and carry no banners. They are pledged to go wherever the weapons are kept and into the corridors of power where decisions are made. The Shambhala warriors have the courage to do this because they know that the dangers threatening life arise from within us. They train in the use of two weapons: compassion for the pain of all, and insight into the interdependence of all.

A new kind of heroic strength awakens by becoming aware of the opponent—oneself—and battling for appropriate care of self and others and for every sort of spiritual advancement. A friend of mine, Sharon, has for many years been a devotee of Sri Chinmoy. This great Indian guru intentionally lived near the home of the United Nations in New York City. Sri Chinmoy worked on all levels, continuously challenging himself with seemingly impossible tasks. When a massively enlightened individual becomes fully engaged in the physical world, amazing events are possible. By the strength of his meditation and steady practice, he attained immeasurable physical powers. He was able to balance a platform on one hand and lift several of his disciples at the same time. This lifting becomes a metaphor for ascending in spiritual development. For many years, he also made a sublime spiritual sport of lifting leaders around the world. He has even been known to lift a small aircraft in which his disciples were about to fly to do good works.

When the disciples of Sri Chinmoy come to him from around the world, they find an important part of their spiritual discipline is physical training. Imbued with spiritual strength, we all have extraordinary capacities latent within us, and under certain conditions are able to perform physical feats we never dreamed possible. More than one mother has lifted a car to save her child. Although Sharon is not a natural athlete, in her twenties she began to participate in the disciplines he recommended. The master sat in the middle of the running track as the disciples ran. Sharon, like many who felt quite weak at first, found after a time that she was capable of running marathons, while others, adept through meditative awareness, have run across deserts or swum back and forth across the English Channel.

SHIELDS, MAGICAL GARMENTS, AND LIES

Extreme challenges and closeness in less supportive circumstances can provoke raging outbursts and allergies. "Don't come near me," scream teenage acne and eczema. "You wouldn't want to touch me!" Under duress, the skin can suddenly stink, bristle like a vicious cat, and harden like a fortress. We may feel swelling within us the mythic power of a god who throws lightning bolts from the sky. To stimulate the external immune system, both male and female warriors often take the time to paint their faces ceremonially as a ritual of protection. Darker impulses in the immune defense system tempt us to respond to hurt by hunting or terrorizing others, to feel the intoxication of violence and the illusion of power, destroying without pity or disgust.

Some regularly use lying as their self-defense or to satisfy their desire for power. Rather than hurling a spear or carrying a shield, a lie becomes lurking armor. Lies provide amusement and lighthearted diversion to idle warriors as they boast of their exploits, like fishermen their fish. A woman confessed to a storytelling group that as a child she lied often to protect herself and to gain support from others. As a more mature adult, she enjoys clowning because everyone knows and accepts the clown's vulnerabilities. As she plays with lies and exaggeration with the freedom of a fool, there are no deep consequences. Like Pinocchio's nose, her lying can be seen.

TALES OF THE CHANGING OF SKINS

Duncan Williamson, the Scots storyteller who grew up among such tales, told multitudes of traditional stories he collected from West Highlanders. Nomadic gypsy families, known in the UK as "travelers," perceive seals as sea-people. Such seals, called "selkies" for their soft, silky coats, may take human form, at least for a time, and entice humans to become seals. Duncan's father would take the bagpipes and walk along the shore playing tunes to the selkies. With their fondness for music and stories, sometimes fifteen or twenty would gather to hear him play. Often in stories and songs about them, selkies do no harm, unless people treat them badly. Then they teach a lesson. Those who are good to them receive goodness in return. The travelers believe that by respecting the selkies they will have a better way of life.

In Duncan Williamson's collection called *The Broonie, Silkies and Fairies* is a tale about a minister on the West Coast of Scotland who hated seals because they broke his nets. One Sunday morning, he killed a wee baby seal that was caught in his net. When his wife became ill and died mysteriously soon after, he advertised for a housekeeper to help with the care of his little girl. A woman soon appeared at his door with long dark hair and the brown eyes of a seal. She was lovely and weirdly quiet, yet his daughter took to her right away. As the story is told, the two spent more and more time on the beach until one day the father stood, aghast, to see them disappear together forever into the water.

Stories from all lands portray the struggles and shifts in the skin. When aggression is called for, mild-mannered Clark Kent, immune system thoroughly aroused, takes on the very physical heroic form of Superman, tough and quick, a man of steel muscles.

TALES OF THE EXTERIOR IMMUNE SYSTEM IN ACTION

As inner battles play out in the world at large, tales tell in story and song the terrible truth of mortal combat. All who love competitive sports sometimes relish in body and soul the crude battle cry, the pagan glee at captured enemy, and the fierce scream of power discharged. The *Iliad,* the Mahabharata, the French saga *The Song of Roland,* and many a modern film depict the chaos of crude, unenlightened "victory," with the warrior hero and the crowd screaming to celebrate war's death and destruction. A traditional English tale highlights how physical closeness can lead to danger.

⚜ ⚜ ⚜

Hanner Dyn

King Arthur in his youth was fond of wrestling, and few dared to challenge him. An old man who had been a champion in years gone by told the young king that his only remaining competitor was one who had tired out all the others. "He, of all wrestlers, is the most formidable. At first you will think him so insignificant as to be hardly worth a contest. But after a while, you will find him growing strong. He seeks out all your weak points as if by magic; he never gives up."

"His name! His name!" said Arthur, eager for the challenge.

"His name is Hanner Dyn. His home is everywhere, but on his own island you will be likely to find him sooner or later. Keep clear of him, or he will get the best of you in the end and make you his slave, as he makes slaves of all whom he has conquered."

The young Arthur searched for Hanner Dyn. He landed at island after island. He saw many weak men who did not dare to wrestle with him, and many strong ones whom he could always throw. One day he came to a far-off island he had never seen before and which seemed uninhabited. Presently, there came out from beneath an arbor of flowers a miniature man, as graceful and quick as an elf.

Arthur eagerly said to him, "Tell me, young man, do you know the whereabouts of Hanner Dyn?"

"I am he," said the laughing little man, taking hold of his hand.

"What do they mean by calling you a wrestler?" asked Arthur.

"Oh," came the coaxing reply, "I *am* a wrestler. Try me."

The king took him and tossed him in the air with his strong arms, till the boy shouted with delight.

He then took Arthur by the hand and led him about the island, showing him his house, gardens, and fields. He showed him the rows of men toiling in the meadows or felling trees. "They all work for me," he said, carelessly. Then the boy led him to the house; he asked Arthur what his favorite fruits and beverages were, and had all at hand. In size and years he seemed a child, but in his activity and agility he was almost a man. When young Arthur told him so, he smiled, as winningly as ever, and said, "That is why they call me Hanner Dyn, the Half-Man." Laughing merrily, he helped Arthur into his boat and bade him farewell, urging him to come again. The king sailed away, looking back on his winsome little playmate with affection.

Many months later Arthur came that way again. Again the merry child met him, having grown a good deal since their earlier meeting. "How is my little wrestler?" asked Arthur.

"Try me," said the boy.

The king tossed him again in his arms, finding the delicate limbs firmer, and the slender body heavier than before, though he was still easily manageable. There were more men working on the island. Arthur noticed that their expressions were not cheerful.

It was, however, a charming sail to the island and thereafter the king often bade his steersman guide his small ship that way. The rapid growth and increased strength of the laughing boy startled him. Arthur and Hanner Dyn wrestled and the king marveled to see how readily the young wrestler caught on to the tricks of the art. Hanner Dyn grew fast into a tall young fellow, still merry and smiling. Instead of the weakness that often comes with rapid growth, his muscles grew ever harder and harder.

One day, in a moment of carelessness as they were wrestling, Arthur received a back fall, but landed on moist ground. Rising with a quick motion, he laughed at the angry faces of his attendants and bade the boy farewell. He noticed the men at work in the fields glancing up, and exchanging looks with one another.

Before long, Arthur revisited the island to teach the saucy youth a lesson. Months had passed, and Hanner Dyn was maturing into a man of princely promise, but with the same sunny look. The youth greeted him joyously. The sullen field hands watched their usual wrestling match. An aged Druid, whom Arthur had brought ashore with him, sat watching.

As the two of them began to wrestle, the king felt, by the very grasp of the youth's arms, by the firm set of his foot upon the turf, that this was to be unlike any previous effort. The wrestlers stood breast to breast, each resting his chin on the other's shoulder. They grasped each other round the body, as each tried to force the other to touch the ground with both shoulders and one hip, or with both hips and one shoulder; or else to compel the other to let go of his hold for an instant. Either of these successes would give the victory. As often as Arthur had wrestled, he never before had been so well matched. The competitors struggled and writhed, half lost their footing and regained it, yet neither yielded. All of Arthur's boatmen refused to believe their eyes, even when they felt their king was in danger. At last, Arthur compelled Hanner Dyn to lose his hold for one instant in the first trial.

The half-blind old Druid, who had been resting, opened his eyes. He himself had been a wrestler in his youth and he called warningly, "Save thyself, O king!"

At this, Arthur again roused his failing strength for the next trial. Gripping his rival round the waist with a mighty grasp, the king raised him bodily from the ground and threw him backward till he fell flat, like a log, while Arthur himself fell fainting. Nor did he recover until he found himself in the boat, his head resting on the knees of the aged Druid.

The old man said to him, "Never again, O king, must you confront the danger you have barely escaped! Had you failed, you would have become the slave to Hanner Dyn, whose strength has been maturing for years to overpower you. If you had yielded, although you are a king, you would have become just another one of those who till his fields and do his bidding. For do you not know what the name 'Hanner Dyn' means? It means 'habit.' A habit, at first weak, then growing constantly stronger, may end in conquering even kings!"

ENLIGHTENING THE SKIN'S AGENDA

Margaret Jones is a prevention specialist in Maine who uses such stories very successfully in her work. Like other social workers who are committed to therapeutic storytelling, she often tells teenagers at risk of substance abuse and other self-damaging habits about a good boy who spotted a small rattlesnake slithering toward him.

> The boy had been warned many times by his grandfather that poisonous fangs could kill him and he started to walk around the snake, but the snake smiled and called out to him. "Would you be so kind as to give me a ride? Look at me. I am such a little snake and you are so big and strong. How could I possibly hurt you? Besides wouldn't you like some company?"
>
> The boy tentatively picked up the snake and let it wrap itself around his shoulders. "Don't worry, my young man, I won't hurt you."
>
> With that, the boy relaxed and even enjoyed the company of the snake. But when the boy bent over to release his traveling companion, the rattlesnake bit him in the neck. The boy, sensing he might not survive, cried, "Why did you bite me? I trusted you! I thought we were friends."
>
> The rattlesnake replied, "It is my nature to bite. You knew that before you carried me." And with that the rattlesnake slithered away without even a second glance at the boy.

Many crudely antisocial heroic activities are immortalized in story and song. In the circa 2000 BC myth, Gilgamesh, the king of Uruk, is intensely physical. With mammoth ego and physical prowess, he wants to stop the flow of time in every combat and become a god. Perverse and single-minded, in his pride he strives for timeless fame. Each of his exploits proves antagonistic to his own community. He takes young warriors to destruction and sleeps with virgins as they are about to wed. He scorns the goddess of love and fertility and oppresses his people by forcing them to build an extravagant wall.

Less egocentric, more blithe myths also portray our exterior immune system's zest for swift and solid victory. In this kind of story, we meet heroes or heroines who, like our modern athletes, have gone through long, steady years of training, and they have attained splendid prowess in both love and war. An old Irish tale tells of the King of Erin who was seeking warriors to defend the shores of Erin and Albion.

> Three of the Fianna warriors eventually came forward: Carnac from Brittany, Tor from Alba, and Quilty from Erin. The High King needed to know how long it would take for each to run to the sands of the north, to the sands of the south, to the sands of the east, and to the sands of the west to see if there were any strange footprints or any stranger to be found on the shores of Erin or Albion. Said Carnac, "I can go from Brian to Cork in three bounds." Tor said he could race on his hands to give the others a fair chance

and take the mountain Ben Bulba at a running leap. He could run as fast as a cat between two houses, faster than it takes for a leaf to leave a tree and touch the ground.

The King of Erin replied, "Not fast enough." Then he turned to Quilty: "How fast can you run?"

"I can run as fast as it takes for a woman to change her mind."

"When will you go?" asked the king.

And Quilty said, "My Lord, I have already returned."

Another Irish myth says of Finn MacCool, the greatest of heroes in the Irish story tradition, that when it came to the training of his men to become the boldest and bravest and swiftest in the land, his athletes underwent a mighty schooling. Finn demanded that all his warriors were as versed in poetry as they were masters of their weapons, to develop their agility and presence of mind. In order to join the mighty band of warriors called the Fianna, young men were tested with only a small shield and a hazel wand for protection. Once that test was passed, the warriors were taken into the forest and their hair was braided and topped with a head scarf. Then they were chased by Fianna warriors. Even if they were not overtaken, if one of the braids of their hair was out of place, they were deemed unfit to join the band. Next each warrior had to jump to the height of his head or run under a wand held at the height of his shin. He failed if he so much as paused in his running, or cracked a dry twig under foot, or bent a blade of grass.

Storytellers in the past—and some still today—were trained in physical prowess. Recounting the physical details of stories can be an athletic feat in itself. Like the Fianna, Turkish storytellers today learn to meet very high standards during their eight-year training. To merit the storytelling medals that blazon their chests, they must master several dozen basic melodies before they begin the craft of speaking stories. In their own language, they learn to make up stories, praises, and insults on the spot, using a strict rhyme scheme and meter when a theme is called out. One of their tests involves their speaking with a double-ended pin placed between their lips. Engaging at least two hundred facial and neck muscles, they can use only words without lip sounds. With this sharp extra challenge, they are disqualified if they draw blood.

MAGICAL GARMENTS AND TRANSFORMATION

The complex responses of the skin's immune system inspire amateur and professional storytellers in many languages. I invited one of my healing story groups to describe their immune response in terms of landscape and architecture. A woman pictured herself as a splendid castle. She sent warning glances to the interior of the castle as an enemy approached. She could lower a luminous bridge for the horses and riders she trained for victory against invaders. If strangers approached, passes closed, outposts and scouts awoke. Her description helped her to gather strength in a difficult time.

The fur of Beauty's Beast and the clammy skin of the Frog Prince cast off reveal noble human beings who are eager for love. By a similar process, Dame Ragnall casts off ugliness and becomes beautiful. As human love transforms the animal body, in countless stories a worthy human gradually or abruptly emerges from an animal skin. In the Grimms' tale called "Allerleirauh," a distraught king insists on marrying his own daughter. He is stirred by violent love for her because she reminds him of his dead wife.

To stall him, the horrified daughter insists that he first provide her with three dresses: one as shining as the sun, one as silvery as the moon, and one as bright as the stars. Then she asks for a mantle made of a thousand different furs sewn together, one of every kind of animal in the kingdom.

The amorous king does not give up and commands the cleverest maidens in his kingdom to weave the dresses. Then he orders his huntsmen to catch one of every kind of animal and take from it a piece of skin. After the many furs have been sewn together into a mantle, the king spreads the coat before his daughter, declaring, "The wedding shall be tomorrow."

The princess nevertheless protects herself. She disguises herself completely in the mantle of furs, blackens her face and hands, and quietly slips out of the castle that night, bringing the three dresses with her concealed in a nut. She walks the whole night until she comes to a great forest and at last finds a hollow tree where she hides herself and falls asleep. Hiding in the hairy mantle inside the hollow tree gives her time to rest from the ordeal with her father. At the end of this tale, the protective husk of the old tree and the fur skins fall away, revealing the celestial radiance of her love for a good prince.

Ancient Mayan culture tells a transformation tale of Xipe Toltec, who was born without any skin at all. The ugliest and poorest of the gods, his flesh hung on his bones in revoltingly smelly lumps. When at last he threw himself into the Sun, he was reborn as the god of spring and flowers. It is said that praise and time itself was born when he arose from his sacrifice to receive his skin.

⋯⋰⋰⋰⋯

TRANSFORMATIONAL STORYTELLING
Skin Affirmation
Humanity shares one sacred skin.

Basic Skin Story Dynamic
Competition becomes companionable athletic vigor.

Skin Protagonists and Antagonists
Skin protagonists (characters who support skin health) are athletic, competitive, and willing to take risks. They sometimes manifest great prowess and inner lightness as they take on

challenges and progress in their chosen sport or other arena of achievement. They bare their skin to manifest their strength and vitality.

Skin antagonists (characters who express skin dysfunction) are stressed and fidgety. They intimidate others with hostile looks and threats. Scolding, sadistic, and demeaning, they hurt others to grab attention and energy as they attack the other's clarity and sense of self. They rupture relationships, even using violence with pleasure to establish their dominance.

Basic Story Elements

Myths and stories often resonate with specific internal processes. This reliable pattern invokes well-being and resilience in every cell of your body:

Setting Out: The protagonist sets out in quest of greater love, strength, justice, wisdom, and happiness.

Trouble: One or more obstacles and/or antagonists interfere with the journey.

Help: Wise and benevolent help comes, often giving a gift.

Positive Ending: The protagonist fulfils the quest with joy and celebration.

SUMMONING YOUR STORYTELLER

Skin-strong storytellers like to feel fit and aglow. Their style of telling displays their physical strength. They enjoy the challenge of bringing a tale to an audience and making physical contact with them. They delight in the sensory richness of the details in their stories: warm and cold, prickly and smooth, hard and soft. They feel daring adventure to the tips of their fingers and toes. As they move inside the power of a tale, they wear skintight clothes and may even enjoy practicing a tale naked. Their voices are robust; their teeth bite into consonants with a metallic ring. They tend to express physical sensations and physical effort in the stories they tell and they love competition. Competing with themselves, they work up a triumphant spirit by contending with a more challenging tale than they did before, or outdoing storytellers who preceded them.

Exercises to Explore and Balance the Skin

Therapeutic touch. How do you take care of your skin? Babies, especially those in intensive care units, do better when they receive massage. This is probably true for all of us. Our lives would be healthier and our immune response would hum pleasantly with regular massages. Describe a massage you have received, or an environment that makes you feel as if you are receiving a splendid massage.

Go barefoot and describe as poetically as you wish the meeting of your skin with the skin of the earth, the skin of the sky, of a tree, or of another person.

A conversation with your skin. Sit down and allow your skin to speak to you. Listen with energetic attention to all that it has to say about its stresses and its needs.

Bumps and bruises. Tell about one of your scars, bumps, or bruises. You survived, with marks to prove it. Touch your skin as your recount this story.

Aggression and tenderness. Make up a brief imaginative tale about an athletic warrior with at least one of the skin protagonist characteristics listed. At first, let aggressive strength prevail and then allow it to blossom into compassion and tender new awareness of the opponent.

Apathy is the result of living in an embattled world and ignoring our own ability to change reality through our own efforts. Like a child, make war paint. Wash and then cover yourself with designs to show your power and courage to face battle, perhaps with arrows and a skull and crossbones. Beat a drum, and tell a small but important tale about harnessing your suppressed anger and winning a battle with the apathy it has created.

The power of music. Attacking notes and whole musical scores, many musicians roll up their sleeves and find release and enjoyment from vigorous practice. Describe an athletic, musician, or another artist or entrepreneur who wrestles to win and won't take "no" for an answer. Describe what results from the battle. When did you last put out strength you did not know was in you during a contest or at another challenging time?

Design a shield. Design a shield. Then tell a story about its protective power, referring to skin protagonist and antagonist characters. Create a story about the loss of this shield, and about finding a different and more wonderful one.

Casting off old skin. It can be empowering to cast off an old skin. What was happening in your life when you wanted to give away your clothes and buy a new outfit? Describe someone, perhaps yourself, who casts off an old skin and outworn habits.

Expanding Skin Awareness Through Dance, Music, and Yoga

Dance
As you clench and relax your fists, feel the gripping and releasing of other muscles throughout your body. Dance as if your lover is a divine wrestling partner.

Suggested music
Tchaikovsky, Dance of the Cossacks from *The Nutcracker Suite*
Prokofiev, Pas de deux, The Montagues and the Capulets, from *Romeo and Juliet*
Beethoven, *Symphony no. 5*
Verdi, *Otello*

Yoga asanas (Sanskrit names in italics)
Child pose *(Balasana)*
Cobra *(Bhujangasana)*
Warrior poses *(Baddha Konasana)*

12

Gentle Judge: The Pericardium

The pericardium, the membranous sac of connective tissue that envelops the heart, is sometimes known as "the heart protector." The tissue of the pericardium is both sensitive and strong. Like other delicately strong tissue that surrounds our organs and holds them in place, it corresponds to supportive linings of all sorts, as in coats, gloves, and old-fashioned bridal hope chests lined with fine fabric. In Chinese medicine, the heart protector meridian begins in the pericardium and descends to the diaphragm to join the skin meridian, its balancing organ. Then it flows up through the armpits and down the inner arms to the elbow creases, through the forearms and palms of the hands, to the tips of the middle fingers.

To sense the subtle strength of your pericardium, place your hands in front of your chest in prayer position. With heels together, straighten your legs and back. As energy stirs in and around the lower spine, the bottom of your rib cage will spring open and forward. When it does, coax your shoulders back and down. Now as you press your palms and fingers together, especially push the length of your middle fingers against one another. As your chest muscles continue to release, breathe broad open breaths into the middle of your palms. You may experience a refreshing sense of calm openness. Perhaps you will feel more centered and less stiff. To experience more fully this energy patterning, reach both hands behind your back. Try putting your palms and fingers together facing upward in prayer position. Then press your hands against the middle of your back. Who does not need prayers behind, in front, and in all directions? As you press your hands against your spine, you may feel a rush of energy moving inward and forward. Now breathe freely and

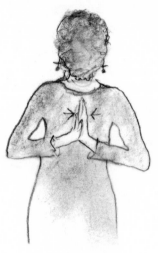

Pericardium Excerise

relax. You might experience an enchanted castle waking, doors unlocking, windows opening in the mind, and fresh winds bringing good news.

When the pericardium is out of balance, limbs and heart feel weak. A woman who attended one of my storytelling as a healing art workshops discovered in the process of creating a story that her pericardium could speak for her, and felt unexpected awe. It was the first spontaneous story she had told in her adult life, and afterward she carefully wrote it down because the images in her story moved her so deeply. When it was time for her to share her story to the group, she read with gleeful amazement:

Once upon a time there lived a man and a woman who wanted very much to have a child. Finally, when they had almost given up, a child came, and they were overjoyed. Soon after the babe was born, however, they were horrified to learn that the infant had been born without any inner protection for her heart. It seemed to them that with such a fearful condition the child would be in danger of dying, but the child did not die. Her heart, however, remained exposed for anyone to see. Her parents dressed her carefully in protective clothing, and never let anyone know of their daughter's vulnerable heart condition. But the child, even beneath the layers of clothing, was finely tuned to the pain and suffering in the world around her. Her heart would become red and throbbing and painful, sometimes swelling and pushing against her clothing. The girl did not know what to do with all the pain she absorbed from others.

One day her godmother came to visit. Seeing the girl's pain, she said, "My goddaughter must go at once to the place of the setting sun, and there she will find help."

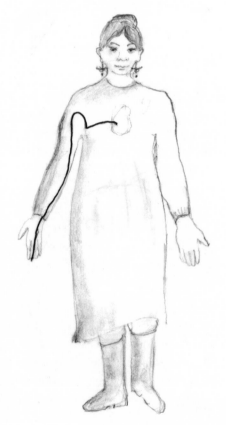

The Pericardium Meridian

So the parents filled a pack with food and clothing for their daughter and with sadness in their hearts sent her off. She walked to the outskirts of the town she had known throughout her childhood and on through the next town and the next. At last she came upon a land that was devastated by drought. All around her people were hungry. Their fear and pain went straight to her heart and she threw herself down into a dry field where she began to cry. As her tears flooded, her cries touched the heart of the sky. Rain poured down on the parched town and the joyful sounds of the townspeople followed the child.

Wandering on, just as she reached another town it began to snow. A man and woman took her into their home, fearing that she would not survive the storm. She slept fitfully. This couple had lost their only child and although they had gone on with their lives, their unexpressed grief hung heavily around them. Sadness filled every corner of the house and quietly entered the girl's heart. It began to throb painfully. Toward dawn, she dreamed of the child who had died. The child spoke to her, begging her to tell the parents that all was well with her, and that she was very near to them. The traveler awakened and told her dream to the couple, who cried out in joy and grief that poured forth in abundant tears. The girl soon went on.

Weary from weeks of journeying, she came at last to the place of the setting sun. In front of her in every direction were trees joined by enormous spiderwebs. The girl trembled and began to turn back the way she had come. But then she remembered her godmother. She faced the horizon. Ahead of her was a vast web that had been woven by a very old spider. Finding her courage, the girl ran straight into this very web. As it covered her body, at first she felt terror. Then she gradually became aware of a wonderful tingling sensation. She threw open her clothing and looked down at her heart. Beneath the web, she watched in amazement as iridescent skin wove closely together and surrounded her heart. Soon she could no longer see her heart, yet she felt its warmth beating beneath this marvelous new iridescence.

The traveler returned home to her parents a different person. She now realized that she could care for others without holding on to their pain, and that she could love and yet protect herself. She became a healer in her town, teaching others to find the strength that allows love to flow freely yet with the wise protection it needs.

The author of this story had tapped unexpectedly into the growing strength of her own pericardium. Several weeks later, she continued to experience relief from the making of her story. Eventually, she felt a strong resolve to apply her imagination to helping others, and realized with joy that she had found a new path forward.

Guardian of Morality

As the pericardium guards and protects the heart, it instills, through a subtle process, an urgent sense of morality. It gives us a sense that the body's highest purpose is to be a temple that upholds the laws of life. A subtle bridge between the heart and all the other organs, the pericardium mobilizes our whole being to insist on fairness and justice. When the heart of life is endangered, minute tears in the fabric of the pericardium call for amends.

As the healthy, supple pericardium safeguards us, it is sensitive to our attitudes and deeds. It awakens curiosity about how the letter and spirit of the law affect the quality of life. From reviewing relationships to scrutinizing investments, it stimulates us to search our souls to discover where we have betrayed our deepest beliefs and resolves, to change our ways, and to urge friends and associates to do the same. Those who play out the role of the pericardium in their lives tend to feel a great responsibility that things go well for everyone. With a solemn sense of purpose, these people are often drawn to careers as public servants. They sit in courtroom, pulpit, school administrators' offices, and abbots' cells; at their best, they may raise a diamond gavel and lower it with hammer-like precision and resolve. They make quietly powerful bureaucrats, inspectors, church prelates, judges, lawyers, and bankers. They are also formidable family members and life coaches. My dentist exemplifies this type. All day long he makes sure his patients understand fully their options and the likely consequences of each.

Opening the Book of Life

One day at the Meridian Stretching Center, several of us were exploring various stretches with Bob Cooley to activate the pericardium energies. After holding a stretch for a few moments, an intensely disciplined lawyer said that he was now acutely aware that he spent his entire days judging others. Totally absorbed in policies, rules, and regulations, he recognized that he normally had very little sense of his personal life. In the mirror, he saw for the first time how pale he was by comparison with others, and realized the tendency for his blood to constrict as he defined abuses and strove to support inner rectitude. While I was resting after some intensive stretching, I, too, discovered new awareness. I suddenly could see with more clarity the positive side of intensely judgmental people. I sensed how their subtle feelers reach out to search for the weak points in others. I could sense how everyone lives in this realm at times, this vast "improvement society," with a pressing organic need and agenda to bring moral principles to life. I accepted as never before this aspect of myself.

Whenever anyone is dishonored or attacked, a response creates slight constrictions in the heart protector, as it searches cellular memory for the sacred statutes that put things right. One day, I unexpectedly experienced this myself. After a session of very concentrated stretching, I went home to rest. I soon awakened and was astonished to see a vision before me. The heart protector appeared as an open book, its golden-edged pages imprinted with great subtlety over immeasurable time. I lay astonished, staring at page upon page, in minuscule typeface—an entablature of spiritual wisdom encoded within me. For a time, this vision of the pericardium shone plainly in my wisdom mind. I was filled with questions: Which comes first? Does the physical pericardium emanate from this living spiritual manual? Do body and soul read from this vast ledger? Is this the Book of Life in which our names are written for eternity?

THE ART AND SCIENCE OF JUDGING

Through stretching exercises, I realized gradually that every courthouse is an outer manifestation of the pericardium in action. Healthy, strong moral fiber builds up a palace of justice in which a judge sits behind a polished brass railing holding a gavel. Behind the judge stacks of books guard essential laws that indicate what to do if they are broken. The court comes to order. "Bring in the accused!" We can truly taste innocence and smell guilt. "This stinks to high heaven" and "I don't like the smell of this" are common sayings in many languages. Whether we are in an actual courtroom or not, the strength of the heart protector's fascia awakens our senses and activates intuitive awareness in body and soul so that, despite the appearance of innocence and of excellent manners and appearance, we can feel the rat in the room. We can taste in conversation or story the sweet clear tang of truth.

When a wise judgment has been spoken, a friendly power rises, lifting veils from the eyes and burdens from heart and soul. A worthy judge delivers even a grim sentence gently, with fine distinctions and gracious conclusions. Each judgment has its own effects. When the punishment truly fits the crime, hope is restored. A sense of wonder and trust return. With right judgment, invisible balance pans shift into horizontal harmony. The guarded heart opens, and the whole body breathes with a sense of rightness and is refreshed. The pleasant ozone of truth sparkles in the air, though some may hunch in their seats as if to hide. Life returns to an original state of innocence and openness.

Judgments gone awry, however, constrict laissez-faire openness. Inner circulations may feel as if they have been corked in an old bottle. Stiff judgments pitch the voice down, and down further. A dysfunctional judge may become fixed on cross-examinations and deliver unhealthy verdicts, like the Grand Poobah in Gilbert and Sullivan's *Mikado*. The judge can dole out dire punishments with violent finality. A gavel can become a sledgehammer with the force of Mars, the god of war, behind it. "Not good enough" may sound like the locking of a very bleak cell, or nails hammering a coffin shut. A name may be stricken from the record.

SHARING THE LIVELY SPIRIT OF THE LAW IN STORIES

Right judgment is stimulated by well-told stories. A sometimes stern tradition of teaching tales exists in many cultures to help listeners develop a sense of right and wrong. These include parables, koans, and fables to guide behavior and to transform disturbing situations and narrow attitudes. Such tales encourage us to imagine consequences and they awaken conscience. Aesop's "The Hare and the Tortoise" teaches that even very slow but steady progress can win the race. South African storyteller Michelle du Toit rewrites one New Testament parable after another into inspired modern-day stories. Parishioners who attend her school of sacred storytelling in Capetown relate these cautionary tales at the altar as part of the holy services. In the following story, a person is very strict toward himself but open toward others.

There was once deep in the woods a hermit who lived a very severe life of fasting, meditation, and prayer. But as much as he was devout and strict with himself, he was also kind to whoever came to his door. It was said that the birds often visited him and occupied his house as their own house, and that the animals came to him as his friend and he would feed the wild things with his own hands.

Tales from many lands tell of the wise judgments of King Solomon. Robert Reiser, a spirited storytelling friend, tells an Ethiopian tale about King Solomon.

❧❧❧❧❧

Josel and the Master Builder

Long ago in old Jerusalem there lived a master builder. He built everything: temples, markets, pyramids, houses for rich and poor. He built his little empire on the principle of economy. If there was one thing Simeon could do, it was cut costs! There he was walking through a building site one evening. He always worked the men as late as he could. By his side walked his assistant, Schmuel. Men cringed from them because when Simeon and Schmuel walked by, jobs were lost.

Suddenly, the master builder's eyes fell on the workmen's fire. "Couldn't the men warm themselves on a fire half that size?" he asked Schmuel.

"Perhaps." Schmuel knew better than to argue with the boss.

"Hey, you!" the master builder shouted at the poor laborer who was warming his hands. "What's your name?"

"Josel, sire."

"Josel, tell me honestly, do you need such a big fire? I bet a strong fellow like you could stand on a mountaintop all night with nothing to warm him."

And so the greedy master builder promised Josel that if he stayed on the mountain all night, without any warmth or protection, he'd get ten aces of farmland and a herd of cattle. On the other hand, if he refused, he'd be out of a job. Josel had no choice but to agree.

Schmuel pulled his boss aside. "You think this is wise?"

The master builder shouted, "If he lives, think of the money I'll save. If he dies... well, one less salary to pay. It's a win-win proposition."

That night Josel told his sad story to his wife. She thought and she thought and suddenly she said, "I've got it. Tomorrow night, husband, I'll build a fire at the foot of the mountain. All night keep your eyes on the fire, think of the warmth, and think of me waiting for you. You can do it."

So the next day poor Josel climbed to the top of the mountain. As the sun set, he took up his position and stood shivering in the wind. Sunset and darkness descended. Far away, down at the bottom of the hill, his wife's fire shone like a bright star in the night. As the hours passed, Josel watched. The wind grew colder. The damp dug into his bones, freezing him to the marrow. But the sight of the fire and the thought of his home and his wife and of his children kept him alive. At last he saw the glow of the sun rising over the horizon. He had survived! He ran down to the office of the master builder, and told his story.

But the master builder took the case to court. At the high court, poor Josel explained how he survived the ordeal.

The master builder, who had slept in a warm bed, was in fine voice. He said confidently, "Your honor, the terms were clear. No fire means no fire!"

And, sadly, the judges agreed. They fined Josel three silver coins for wasting their time.

As Josel and his wife left the court, however, a strange hooded figure approached them. "Don't be discouraged. I promise you, justice will be done." And then he vanished.

The next morning a royal messenger pounded on Josel's door. "You are invited to the grand hall of the palace for a special feast in honor of the great judges who serve on our court."

Dressed in their shabby clothing, Josel and his wife stood in the palace ballroom. The royal crier announced from the front of the room: "The feast shall begin as soon as the lamb is cooked!" Again and again the music played, but still there was no food. Soon the guests began to grumble. "Enough!" shouted the judges. They all trooped down to the royal kitchens. On one side of the room stood a beautiful rack of lamb. On the other side of the kitchen blazed a fire. In the middle, his back to them, stood the royal chef.

The master builder sputtered, "What kind of a way is this to cook a lamb? It won't even get warm."

"No, it won't." The chef turned around. It was King Solomon. "It will get no warmer than a man would, watching it from the top of a mountain."

The judges stared at the fire, then they looked at Josel. Then they turned to King Solomon. "Your highness is right. The letter of the law is not always the same as the spirit of the law." Then they turned to the master builder as they pronounced a new sentence. "Give the man his land."

And with that, the feast began.

⋯⋯⋯

New Laws from a Compassionate Heart

In difficult times, the pericardium tends to stiffen. As it gathers and toughens to protect the heart's emotional and physical vulnerability, it constricts the heart's warm healthy circulation. This in turn can lead to stiffness of body and soul. The following story from the island of Haiti exemplifies the relieving power of justice that a story can provide.

⋯⋯⋯

Ay, Ay, Ay

An orphan boy lived with his aunt. No matter how hard he performed the household chores, she always found an excuse to beat him. One day she couldn't find any fault to punish him for, so she sent him to the market to get a whole list of things and told him that if he didn't come home with everything on the list, including some "Ay Ay Ay," she would beat him. He asked her what she meant by "Ay Ay Ay," but all she said was, "People are always saying 'Ay Ay Ay,' and you don't know what it is? Get me some from the market."

The boy left the house crying, and met an old woman. She took him to the river. She helped him catch crabs and then gather pine needles and put them at the bottom of his sack. Then she told him to go to the market for everything else he needed. "When you get home," she said, "when your aunt asks for 'Ay Ay Ay,' tell her to reach deep into the bottom of the sack and she will find it."

The boy did as he was told and went home.

The aunt reached into the sack. The crabs pinched her fingers. The pine needles poked her. She started jumping up and down, crying 'Ay, Ay, Ay!' She made so much noise the neighbors came. Even the sheriff came. When they heard the story, she was forced to stop mistreating the little boy forever.

⋯⋯⋯

Opening the Heart

Thich Nhat Hanh portrayed the unfolding of moral wisdom of the Buddha in his book *White Cloud*. Hermann Hesse, in his book *Siddhartha,* also described the early years of the Buddha as the privileged Prince Siddhartha in his parents' protected and luxurious palaces. As the young Buddha approached his adult years and he began to realize the greatness of wisdom within him as his heart matured. A fuller spectrum of life began to dawn upon him, and he embraced a far more inclusive path of morality than his parents had envisioned for him.

After hearing how young Siddhartha eventually became an enlightened spiritual guide for countless souls, a group of parents who met in a storytelling circle described first leaving home. One young mother said that her parents always looked for the best and showed warm support- ive interest whatever she did and wherever she went. Another wondered with annoyance if she would ever emerge from the atmosphere of her parents' judgmental attitudes. "To this day they constantly look for what is not right in my life," she complained. "They fixate on trouble and have so little pleasure." This woman was exhausted by the effects of the tense pericardium atmosphere of her childhood. As her parents brooded on things not up to par, no one in the family was able to feel relaxed so they never experienced heartfelt enthusiasm and self-acceptance.

Many go about our lives carrying undeserved sentences from childhood. Yet the strong moral fiber of the pericardium, at its finest, makes a shining palace of justice to which our deeds and thoughts willingly go for balanced, fair judgments. A healthy pericardium supports and generates respect for each aspect of life. Great moral leaders such as Mahatma Gandhi and Martin Luther King Jr. recognized that the principles of justice require us to treat the claims of all in an impartial manner, respecting the basic dignity of each individual. Tales from all lands, like this one from Japan, uphold the universal principles of justice that guide us toward decisions based on equal respect for all.

⁓⁂⁓⁂⁓

The Golden Seed

There was once a poor and hungry man who stole a piece of fruit in the marketplace. The vendor had him arrested and brought before the ruling magistrate.

The thief said in his own defense, "If you will pardon me, I will give you a wonder- ful gift."

The magistrate replied gruffly, "What could you have that would seal this bargain?"

The thief took a small seed from his pocket. "When this is planted, it will bear fruit overnight.

It will bear fruit of gold."

So the magistrate insisted that he plant the seed.

"I cannot," said the poor man. "It can only be planted by someone who has never stolen, cheated, or lied. Sir, you have the honor of planting the seed."

The chief magistrate stammered and muttered, "I do not plant crops. Give the seed to my chief prelate."

That prelate refused, saying, "I do not have a green thumb. Give the seed to the Com- missioner of Oaths."

One by one, all the officials in the court refused to plant the seed. Everyone stood in silence.

Finally, the thief said, "Am I to be punished for stealing one piece of fruit when I was hungry, when not one of you is able to plant this seed? Is that justice?"

The magistrate set him free.

⋯⋰⋯⋰⋯

The pericardium helps us on the noble path to right relationships, lifting us beyond petty self-judgment into the much more inclusive wisdom mind. Stories about enlightened beings often intentionally disturb our sense of morality. Sometimes it takes a long time to test out the truth in the story that challenges our sense of justice. As the pericardium quietly protects and upholds the core of life, it can summon a gentle and majestic angel in a helmet, a white knight in shining armor following divine orders, or a gathering of troops in defense of pure justice. With gentle determination, it can lead us to an altar of infinite forgiveness. "Lord, forgive them for they know not what they do" is the other side of the judge's stern attitude that everyone should by birthright know the highest laws of life, keep to them, and thus avoid trouble.

Soon after the events of 9/11 in New York City, Karen, a mother who had learned to apply principles of storytelling as a healing art, told her daughter a story that helped them both experience a sublime court of law. That morning her six-year-old child had told her a dream: "I was on a ship and it crashed. There were a lot of skeletons around and then some people came who were trying to kill us."

Greatly dismayed at first, after a while the mother was able to summon her new authority as a storyteller. She said to her child with quiet confidence, "That sounds like the beginning of a story. It just isn't finished yet." Soon they were snuggling together, as they had done many times before. Not knowing how the story would develop, the mother began speaking carefully nevertheless, trusting that a spiritual process would inspire her words and imagination, and this story emerged.

⋯⋰⋯⋰⋯

The Island of Bones

Once upon a time there were fifteen hundred people on a big strong ship. They sailed out into the ocean with great hope and courage, and sailed on very well, until one day a storm came. The sky darkened and the ocean swelled higher and higher. Up and down the sea tossed the boat as the rain poured and the thunder roared and the winds howled. The people on the boat looked out, but couldn't see what was ahead of them or what was behind them. They were lost, and the ship was tossed here and there. At last it crashed hard into a rock and the boat broke apart. The people swam and tried to hold on to bits and pieces of the boat. They tried to help each other, but the stormy sea kept them going under and coming back up, until they also crashed into the rock. And there they saw skeletons. They also saw a band of pirates who came toward them with daggers in their hands. The good people of the ship feared that the pirates would kill them. This was the island made of bones. The pirates wanted to use their skeletons as landfill. They wanted to kill the good people and have more and more bones.

Suddenly, out of the sky there came another ship, a ship that needed no water. Guiding the ship was an enormous angel with tremendous power. The angel sent a bolt of lightning that stunned and punished the pirates so they could kill no more. Then it gathered the people of the ship. Some of them it brought to Heaven so that they could be made ready to serve Earth. Others it brought to different places all over the world to spread the power of peace.

⋯⋰⋱⋯

The story accepted the child's fears. It depicted fearful events while also acknowledging vastly creative and benevolent spiritual dimensions of life. As her story finished, the mother's imagination suggested that troubles are not endless and that mysterious justice is at work. It portrayed horrifying events transformed mysteriously into wholeness and goodness by higher courts than human ones. Karen guided the story toward the heart of happiness. The child's nightmare became an opportunity for both mother and child to experience comforting wisdom. Karen's daughter pondered the story, was satisfied, and afterward played peacefully with her friends.

Transformational Storytelling

Pericardium Affirmation

I live compassionately, without blame.

Basic Pericardium Story Dynamic

Condemnation becomes informed compassion.

Pericardium Protagonists and Antagonists

Pericardium protagonists (characters who support pericardium health) are candid, impartial mediators who base relationships on a sense of balanced fairness. They are outstandingly as good as their word. They appreciate structure, one thing at a time, and ceremonious habits. They feel open and embracing and are natural philanthropists.

Pericardium antagonists (characters who express pericardium dysfunction) are closed-minded, arrogant, stiff, and shaming. They undermine pleasurable experiences and, although they want to be loved, tend to be masochistic, inciting rejection from others.

Basic Story Elements

Myths and stories often resonate with specific internal processes. This reliable pattern invokes well-being and resilience in every cell of your body:

Setting Out: The protagonist sets out in quest of greater love, strength, justice, wisdom, and happiness.

Trouble: One or more obstacles and/or antagonists interfere with the journey.

Help: Wise and benevolent help comes, often giving a gift.

Positive Ending: The protagonist comes through with joy and celebration.

SUMMONING YOUR STORYTELLER

Storytellers who are strong in the realm of the pericardium come before an audience to bring a sense of what is fair and just, and to expose error. As they seek to align their audience with the forces of justice, their voices embody wise neutrality, free of emotion. They choose stories about how people live and how we should behave according to the immutable and necessary laws of life. Their gestures tend to be ceremonious and exacting as they serve both the letter and the spirit of the law. They speak with equilibrium, uprightness, and solid deliberation, as if behind them is a library of law books, and in their hand a gavel. They are an open book, impartial, and fair, and share humor that brings balance and restores good judgment.

Exercises to Explore and Balance the Pericardium

A tale for the pericardium. Make up a story that includes a pericardium protagonist and antagonist, as described.

Here comes the judge. Laughter lightens a heavy sense of guilt. Imagine you are clothed in a robe of judgment. You carry in your pocket a vial of the oil of mercy. Put on an imaginary or authentic curled white wig and take a high seat above table height. Call to mind a judgment on your life or someone else's. Now imagine that a guinea pig, puppy, and/or other affectionate creatures are called to witness on your behalf. What would they say in your defense? What secret evidence might they surprisingly bring to light?

Judgment Day. Listen to the "Dies Irae" section of Mozart's *Requiem*. It is the Last Judgment, and you are on jury duty. How do you feel about this task? Who is on trial?

A new view of an old sentence. A judge can be stiff and cold when the power of judgment constricts flowing warmth of heart. Let this cold-hearted judge and critic have a holiday, and invite a more malleable judge to the bench. A healthy pericardium is pliable, yet attuned to the laws of life as it helps infinitely powerful wisdom hidden within us inform us how and when to make amends for misdeeds, how to cultivate faith in a lawful universe, and how to forgive. It recognizes different viewpoints and opinions. Stand before yourself with the inner tranquility of a wise judge. Tell about a time when you, or someone close to you, was unfairly judged and thrown into a proverbial dungeon. Look for a much larger picture than you have seen in the past, and deliver a fairer judgment.

Speaking wise judgment. In his autobiography, Gandhi wrote: "To slight a single human being is to slight not only that being, but with him the whole world." Stand with one foot slightly forward. Speak these words aloud in different moods: with a heavy moral tone, a delicate light touch, from a cold viewpoint, and with warmth of heart. As you listen to each tone of voice, notice, for example, that words empty of compassion have a dull metallic sound.

Using the prompt of a nightmare. Any disturbing fragment of a dream or nightmare can be brought to a higher perspective and equanimity through imagery that is in touch with pericardium wisdom. You can trust your imagination and intuition to develop your dream into a story, no matter what fears or doubts you might have about your own creativity and abilities as a storyteller. Accepting the dream, think globally and as if you are listening to a great storyteller who is in touch with the highest spiritual laws. Accept any and all of the images that come to you.

Balancing skin and pericardium. Review the virtues of the skin realm with its earthy, athletic striving. Compare the natural themes of the skin with the pericardium's love of fairness and justice. Imagine partners from each of these two realms who wish to marry one another. What different wedding vows would each one say to the other. Prepare for hilarity as you write out the vows and imagine and/or enact their wedding ceremony.

EXPANDING PERICARDIUM AWARENESS THROUGH DANCE, MUSIC, AND YOGA

Dance

Stand with your hands in prayer position pressed against your heart. Walk judiciously, your forehead upright. Align yourself vertically and horizontally through your shoulders, hips, and knees. Keeping your hands pressed together, go forward, holding your center, calmly balancing each step you take, as if you have weighing pans on either side of your body. Move in a stately dance, as if you have a sword of truth between your hands.

Music

Bach, Cantata no. 140 Sleepers Awake, Sonata no. 2 Sarabande
Friedel Kloke-Eibl, *Meditation des Tanzes*
Mozart, *Requiem*

Yoga asanas (Sanskrit names in italics)

Triangle *(Trikanasana)*
Crow *(Bakasana)*
Standing Forward Bend with hands in prayer position behind back *(Parshvottanasana)*

13

Bountiful Healer: The Thymus

When my spirits were low one day, I went for a walk with a wise friend. He put his arm around me and with every step began to thump on his chest and shout a loud "Ho!" Soon I was tapping on my breastbone and shouting "Ho!" along with him. Fresh energy coursed through us. A new spring came into my steps, as everything around us seemed to be suddenly burgeoning with life.

Tarzan, the famous ape-man in the old movie by that name, beat often on his thymus to celebrate life, and to summon his beloved Jane. Try beating upon this small drumming place at the top of the breastbone, near the lungs and heart. It can be a grand experience to release its fountain of glandular vitality and lymphatic flow. To find fresh zest for life, step forward, and with each breast-beat and footfall, shout through the bountiful jungle of your body and imagination a resounding "Ho!"

According to traditional Chinese medicine, one of the regulatory channels that helps us to breathe and move in harmony with our environment circles the waist, dipping across the abdomen as it pushes the chest up and forward. It is connected with thymus health as it regulates our "gut-level" feelings. A widespread fashion trend lowers the waistline to the belt meridian, exposing the belly. In our increasingly heady and nerve-wrought world, baring the abdomen awakens earthy physical vitality in young and old alike. Traditional wedding gowns are often designed to follow this meridian line, the silk gathered gracefully in a new-moon curve at the belly. Boys enjoying the practice of judo will tie their belts along this line as they prepare to meet life.

When your immune system detects any threat to your survival, an internal attack system goes into action. Any worn-out or unhealthy part of the body attracts the immune system. It detects and acts. It constantly checks the digestive tract, lungs, blood, and virtually every cell of the body to break spells of illness and to heal injuries. It is alert to the effects of alcohol, tobacco, and drugs. Contending with high cholesterol levels, excessive sugar consumption, chemical exposure, food additives, and every sort of new and ancient stress, the immune response can become exhausted, and strategize with the rest of the body to obtain needed rest and repair.

Researchers claim that the thymus is the master gland of the whole immune system, in perpetual training to neutralize or destroy whatever might harm our physical health. Thymus immune activity coordinates with many different organs, tissues, cells, and fluids located throughout the body.

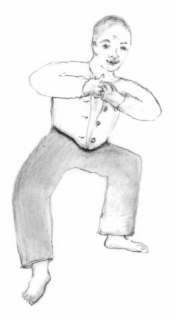

Thymus Exercise

The physiology of immune cells fills volumes of medical books. Countless regenerating white blood cells that contribute crucial balance to the immune system originate in the bone marrow. Approximately half of them go directly into the bloodstream and tissue fluids, but the rest pass through the thymus. These specialized lymphocytes carry out defensive functions. Each immune cell that originates in the thymus, called a T cell, is meticulously programmed for release into the bloodstream on search and destroy missions. These cells go out in clusters and operate with aggressive cunning. They are carried in lymphatic fluids and distributed through vessels, ducts, and lymph nodes. Scientists continue to study with awe their life forces as they survey, destroy, neutralize, and eliminate disease-creating microorganisms.

Fountain of Youth

Ancient Greeks thought of the thymus as the seat of the soul. Throughout our lives, the thymus gland supports our sense of physical abundance and well-being. Researchers continue

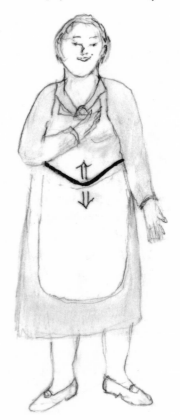

The Belt Channel

exploring how to tap its secrets for health. The thymus gland has an especially mighty mission to protect children. It is about ten times larger at birth than at any other time in our lives. The entire endocrine system changes during adolescence. As the body evolves a mature and more complex immune system, the thymus shrinks gradually to the size of a pea. This shrinkage leads to reduced T-cell activity. The sex hormones that flood the body at puberty impel the thymus to shrink. This has given medical researchers the idea of blocking sex hormones in adult medical emergencies to encourage the thymus to grow again so that it might pump out the large number of T cells it once did.

The whole body is invited by the thymus to the celebration of life. Especially healthy thymus function produces people with gleaming physical health and with natural healing abilities, who generate confidence in the body's abundant generosity. It is a magical provider of energy that puts things right, as the elves do in "The Shoemaker and the Elves" in the Brothers Grimm collection. Those who live in its power seek bountiful physical health for themselves and others. Like Old King Cole and jolly Santa Claus, thymus-strong people tend to be magnanimous to everybody as they strive to make the material world a place of comfort and health for all. Such people bring balance to the apocalyptic, shape-shifting, lean appendix type (see chapter 14).

Wherever they find themselves, thymus-strong folk strive to live well, even if it is from behind the scenes in soup kitchens, or working to provide sumptuous banquets for both rich and poor. Although they embody charismatic powers, they do not especially care to draw attention to themselves, when from their silent posts they bring about hugely gratifying celebrations of life. With their overwhelming generosity, they may be venture capitalists who want to have in order to be able to give. When they farm, they provide abundantly for themselves and others; they may set up food markets rich in fruits and vegetables or gorgeous restaurants stocked with every good comestible, cooking pot, and utensil. As massage therapists and health practitioners, they purvey plant medicine to improve thymus function, such as echinacea, garlic, and sage, or remedies made from the thymus glands of young animals. In touch with needs on a nonverbal, physical level, using the few words they do mainly to stimulate physical action, many teach physical education or practice physical therapy. With a "Ho! Ho Ho!" they tend to celebrate long and often, inviting even beggars to the wedding feast.

Attractive thymus-strong people can activate an irresistible longing in others to be with them. Ted runs a restaurant and in his remaining time is a massage therapist. People flock to his place and tend to stay late and long; his food and massage treatments help them flow and glow with well-being. In his domain, they feel abundantly well taken care of. Whoever is near him feels a mesmeric bonding with the profound glandular strength that causes his neck and eyes sometimes to weave back and forth with a subtle snakelike motion. Yet Ted has difficulty figuring out how to communicate sexually in personal relationships. Physically robust, he easily feels out of touch with his thoughts and his emotions. Like the enchanted prince in the classic tale "Beauty and the Beast," he often feels more secure working invisibly from behind the scenes to be sure his clientele are provided for.

EAT AND TELL STORIES

When two of my dear friends were married, a thymus mood prevailed. It seemed the whole town came to the reception. Round tables on a sunny deck were laden with breads and grains, fruits of every color and shape, bowls of appetizing vegetables, cooked and raw, in glorious combinations. Though every taste bud was honored, the feasting inspired not greed but well-being. Fabulous flowers were set out everywhere. Musicians and storytellers gave their gifts freely, and everyone danced, sang, and feasted for hours.

Bob Kanegis and Liz Mangual, a storytelling and social worker team in Santa Fe, New Mexico, stimulate thymus activity within the whole body of their community. Through an alternatives to violence program, they host a series called FEAST, which stands for Families Eating and Storytelling Together. Local farmers and restauranteurs who enjoy supporting family events that celebrate people eating good food together donate all the food for these events.

A thymus mood of flowing abundance permeates the FEAST community celebrations. By the time these annual events roll around, Bob and Liz have succeeded in building a feeling of community warmth and well-being, and family service agencies have given away most of the tickets. As a labor of love, Bob and Liz speak with many people in advance to ensure that they will feel comfortable when they arrive. The events are accessible to all, old and young, across cultures and economic lines. Liz reports, "We have preschoolers from small, mostly Hispanic towns, Native American teenagers from a Santa Fe residential program, Big Brothers and Sisters, the Boys' and Girls' Club, Girls Inc., the Family Counseling Center, librarians from several towns, and homeschoolers."

Hundreds of people show up for each FEAST event. The format is stories and music, then a community meal, then more stories and music, provided by anyone in the community who wants to share a tale or a song. On one occasion, an elderly Lakota storyteller, historian, linguist, and civil rights activist told stories. Another elder wearing a sequined jacket brought her accordion and a bag of chilies, regaling folks with old-time New Mexico mountain music, accompanied by a guitarist, who knew just how to coax little anecdotes from her. This pair threw chilies to the audience between numbers.

Imbuing their cherished values with humor, other storytellers tell spellbinding personal tales, perhaps about being sent away to a boarding school that lacked indoor plumbing or losing their native language and committing themselves to relearning it. Many bring their children and their parents as well as their grandparents, who also reminisce about bygone days. At these events, everyone learns something new about a family member or friend, and meets and talks with someone they didn't know before. Children demonstrate touching their noses with their toes. Everyone wins something during the raffle of beautiful objects and books donated by some of the native people.

STORIES STIMULATE A SENSE OF ABUNDANCE AND CELEBRATION

Life in all cultures calls for stories that encourage us to transform alienation and disappointment. The Norwegian story "The White Bear King Valemon" tells of a heroine who has lost everything dear to her.

Eventually, she comes to four magical cottages. In the first cottage, she discovers a flask that provides whatever drink she desires. In the second, she finds golden scissors that provide her with any garment she needs. In the third, there is a magical cloth; whenever it is spread, it provides food aplenty. All these gifts she puts to good use. In the fourth cottage, she meets a blacksmith and his wife and their starving, ragged children. She provides for them abundantly before going on to dangerous circumstances, which she navigates successfully.

The following well-known Jewish teaching tale expresses a similar theme.

The Bountiful King

A king who ruled a troubled realm longed bitterly for a child. One day an old wise woman came to the king and queen and proclaimed that a child could be theirs if the king would perform one task. "Your Majesty, use your army to dispose of all the human waste that creates sickness in the land. Dig canals so that the waste may go to one place and water for drinking and cooking to another." And soon the pestilence that had afflicted the people for many years was gone. But as no child was conceived, the king summoned the old woman to the throne room.

"Oh, King, now parcel out the land to the serfs and peasants, and allow each family enough for a bounteous life."

"Why should I give what is mine?" asked the king. But the promise of a child of his own spurred him to give every peasant and serf his own land.

Still no child was conceived, and in his wrath the king condemned the old woman to death.

"Your Majesty, you may kill me. But one last requirement will bring fruit, of this I am sure. The last thing you must do is dismantle your army. For decades our kingdom has fought war after war. Make good treaties with your neighbors."

The king longed for a child so desperately that, against his better judgment, he did as she asked. And so for the first time in memory there were no armed guards. Children danced safely at the borders. But after a year, when again no child had been conceived, the king summoned the old woman to the scaffold to die.

But she spoke quietly to him. "You have given your people health. You have given them wealth, and the security of peace. Your name always will be spoken with honor through the generations. You will be remembered by all the children of this land."

And the king took her hand as he gazed at the bounteous landscape he had created, and knew that what she said was true. Because of her, his actions had given birth to a greater life that he had ever dreamed possible.

⁓✲⁓✲⁓✲⁓

In stories, as in life, festivals and feasting can last for many days and nights. Herman Ostermann in *The Alaskan Eskimos* recounts a story about a man and a woman who lived near the sea.

⁓✲⁓✲⁓✲⁓

The House of Celebration

A lonely couple had a son, and when he was a young boy, his father made a bow for him. Soon he was hunting skillfully, but one day he did not return from his day of hunting. His parents searched for him in vain.

They conceived another child, another son. He too became a skilled hunter, and one day he too did not return. The man and the woman's hearts ached. Then they conceived and the wife bore a third son. When he went hunting deep in the forest, he saw a young eagle circling in the sky. He thought of shooting it, but before the thought reached his hands, the eagle landed near him. The eagle pushed back his hood and revealed the face of a powerful young man. Young Eagle Man spoke: "Unless you give a song feast, you shall die. Tell me, do you promise, or do you not?"

The third son replied, "I know not what a song feast is. Tell me about song. Speak to me about feast."

The Eagle Man spoke: "Will you or will you not?"

And the third son agreed to what he did not know.

Then Eagle Man spoke again: "Come with me and meet my mother. She will teach you what you do not know. When you have grasped how to give birth to a song that becomes its own singing, when you know the joy that dances its own dance, you may freely return home to your parents."

They traveled toward the high mountains. They traveled a long, long way. At last they came to a great mountain, which they climbed. After a time of climbing, the young hunter heard a strange pounding sound. It grew louder and louder.

Eagle Man asked, "Do you hear? It is the mother's heartbeat."

Then they came to Eagle Man's dwelling. He invited the young hunter to come and meet Eagle Mother. Eagle Mother sat alone on a wooden platform at the sky's edge with ragged feathers; she was deeply worn with age and sorrow.

"Mother, this young hunter has promised that he will hold a song feast when he returns home. Yet he knows nothing about beating a drum. Mother, this hunter has come to be with us, and to learn."

Upon hearing her son's words, a new light came into Eagle Mother's face. She thanked the young hunter, saying, "First you must build a House of Celebration so that people may gather in one place."

So the two young men set about building a House of Celebration. Then Eagle Mother showed them how to make the ordinary drum and the festivity drum, and to listen for the heartbeat of sky and earth, or wind and water. Then she led them to the knowing that helps words become songs, and songs become their own singing. She helped them beat the drums when singing arises; and she taught the dance that joy dances.

When they could do it all and knew it well, Eagle Mother spoke: "Return to your home and build a Festival House. Create songs. Then gather food in abundance and call your people and hold a song feast."

The young hunter replied, "But we know no one. We live at the edge of the dark sea and the dark forest. We know no one but ourselves."

The mother then opened his vision, and soon she sent him home to his parents. He explained to them what he had learned: "Human people live alone because we do not know the sacred gift of Celebration."

In the days and weeks that followed, his parents came with him and they chose a place and together built a House of Celebration. They hunted until there was food in abundance. They helped words become songs, and they listened for the songs to become their own singing. They made drums and beat them, until they knew how to beat drums. They danced with joy. They sang to their words and to the beating of the drums.

When all was prepared, the young hunter went into the forest, climbed hills and mountains, and searched for guests along rivers and streams to the ocean's edge. As Eagle Mother had promised, he met people in ones and twos. Some had the skin of wolves, others the skin of caribou and fox. He invited them all. His brothers' spirits accompanied him, and together they made a song feast. The old father beat the festival drum, deep and resonant like Eagle Mother's heart. All learned and sang and danced until dawn, their feet beating the earth and their voices like wings beating on the night skies.

Only at dawn did the guests make ready to leave the new House of Celebration. They fell onto their paws, they dove into the great oceans and rivers, they lifted into the skies, and the parents and their son knew for the first time who their guests had been, for such are the powers of celebration.

Time passed and again the young hunter was deep in the forest. Again he met Eagle Man and together they made their way to the faraway great mountain. Old Eagle Mother wanted to see the young hunter, who had been true to his word and had begun to give humankind the song feast. When they came to the top of the mountain, Eagle Mother rose and stepped forward to greet the young hunter. By the power of celebration, she had become fresh and strong again.

ⁿ⚬ⁿ⚬ⁿ⚬ⁿ

THE TRANSFORMING ADOLESCENT THYMUS IN STORY

The house of celebration is the body. It takes time for adolescents to build this foundation. They must learn the ways of the drum, which beats their vital inner circulations into strong rhythmic patterns. They must learn to be present to themselves and others, and to dance with animal vitality.

As growing teenagers build their bodily house of celebration, a life and death struggle is occurring within them. They must transform their former child bodies into unfamiliar new ones. Who has not felt both deeply entranced and repelled by teenagers as the endocrine system activates simultaneously the power of death and of procreation? Without the skills and the spirit of celebration, frustrated desire awakens destructive impulses. During these times, many youngsters feel compelled to withdraw into dark fantasies and long spells of privacy and sleeping. As in the wise old fairy tale "Sleeping Beauty," no one must enter their thorny walled garden, "on pain of death."

The right words and plotline can set off healthy thymus activity and support immune function throughout the body. By nourishing a healthy felt sense of abundance and celebration of life, a good story can show a path to rebuilding devastated immune function. Oscar Wilde's "The Selfish Giant" depicts this profound power of renewal. In the story, a giant ogre returns home after seven years away. Like an adolescent feeling too awkward and defensive to celebrate life, he chases away all the children who love to play in his garden and builds a high wall to keep them out. When spring comes that year to the giant's garden, birds do not sing and the trees forget to blossom. Yet one morning the giant discovers the children have crept through a little hole in the wall, and are sitting in every tree. Like thymus rebalancing the whole endocrine system, the trees fill themselves with blossoms and rejoice with the return of the children. Only one of the trees is still covered with frost and snow and a child is trying to climb into its branches. So moved is the ogre at the sight of this blessed child that he reaches down, picks up the boy, and gently puts him into the tree, which blossoms in response to his gentle deed. Soon afterward the ogre demolishes the wall he had built around his garden, and bounteously welcomes the children to play again in his garden. Many years thus pass happily in the giant's garden until on his death day he himself is welcomed into the Garden of Paradise.

PICTURING THE THYMUS GLAND'S MESMERIC MIGHT

When the clandestine dramas of the internal immune system surface in stories, as in life, their energies can sometimes cast very dark shadows. Within these shadows lurk many who are unable to give love or to feel it within themselves. Instead they envelop us in a mesmeric mood of envy and material comfort and ease. With advertising schemes and markets of fascinating items, or restaurants with mindlessly abundant cuisine and entertainment, they may impel us into their power, until, like them, we lose touch with our souls and rational discernment.

This threatening side of thymus immune activity was portrayed in Homer's great epic when Odysseus was temporarily blown off course on his homeward journey and landed on the isle of the Lotus-Eaters. The moment his fellow sailors went ashore, they were attracted to a strange plant. As soon as they ate of this "lotus," an ominous euphoria overcame them and they forgot their past and their mission. As they lived in bondage to a continual feast of addictive plants, they disconnected entirely from their former selves. Odysseus had to force them back on board his ship from that hypnotic land; he tied them up until they were safely away.

Great stories encode personality patterns in picture language. The dark side of thymus activity acts like a snake that is freezing a field mouse for capture. People in its power may create idyllic places to which others must come on their terms. With mesmeric gazes, they demand cooperation. The sensible thoughts and moral constraints of others easily dissolve in their presence because, perhaps unconscious of their own power, they are adept at the brainwashing techniques that lead to submission, childlike obedience, and compliance.

Joseph Campbell often warned us that when we neglect stories, they cannot give us their wisdom and perspective. From them, we can glean insight into ourselves and others as we awaken and see more clearly. The main characters in "King Midas" and "The Emperor Has No Clothes" captivate everyone into a trance that binds them into their physical reality. The ugly queen captures Snow White into her spell. Rip Van Winkle wanders in the mountains and finds himself mesmerized for long years by the hospitality of "little men," just as Thomas the Rhymer, a Scots-Irish traditional figure, is mesmerized into a faery realm.

The immune defense system under the influence of an overstimulated thymus gland can cause great destruction. Muscles on high alert may puff like adders to strike—ominous arousal that is woeful to witness or to embody, a primal force without ethical awareness. In stories and in life, crazed and wounded animals and mesmeric mythical monsters roam with huge physical energy. If others have what they want, out of raging envy they may set out to trash their world. All of Ireland knows tales of how Finn McCool became captain of the mighty warrior band called the Fianna, and how unearthly music that came to Tara, their meeting hall, put them into deep trance.

Then an appalling monster would come and wreck havoc on Tara. Each time this mesmeric music sounded, Finn McCool was the only man amongst them who could resist the charismatic trance cast by this monster, and so defeat it. Beowulf , another ancient hero, vanquished similarly mesmeric and murderous fiends.

A Jewish teaching tale called "The Desert Island" exemplifies the dynamics of healthy and unhealthy thymus activity. The story moves through isles where all things are mysteriously provided. The wealthy father in this story creates for himself and his son an oasis that holds everything for their mutual happiness.

> When the boy comes of age, his father provides a fine ship for him with everything he needs to sail proudly onward to seek his own life. Eventually, the ship is lost in a violent storm, and only the young man survives the destruction. He lands on a shore and experiences a new realm of dazzling abundance. Yet he notices an ominous undercurrent on this strange island of abundance. A company of celebrating people meet and accompany him in a splendid carriage to a palace in the center of their city. They crown him king, and tell him he will only be king for one year. After that he will be put on a boat and sent to a particular desert island. Then they surround him with admiration and love. Every official approves of him, and the people offer praises and give him unquestioning obedience. With ample yet oddly impersonal sensual delight, all his desires are immediately met in this realm. He sees no misery or aging anywhere. After drifting in kingly abundance at first, he begins to question. Everyone evades the young man's questions until at last an old man tells him how to break the spell of this strange paradise, and the resourceful young man goes about doing for himself what his father had done for him. He equips a boat with building materials and provisions and begins to build up a place on another island, in readiness for the time when his weird reign will end. Thus he is able to sail away to build a life that includes consciousness, history, and the promise of a healthy, safe, and generous old age.

Transformational Storytelling

Thymus Affirmation

My life is a bounteous celebration.

Basic Thymus Story Dynamic

Destructiveness transforms into caring, abundant generosity.

Thymus Protagonists and Antagonists

Thymus protagonists (characters who support thymus health) are in touch with the physical flow of life. They delight in opulence and the restoration of the body to its natural health. They are vigorous and warmly hospitable hunters, providers, and healers.

Thymus antagonists (characters who express thymus dysfunction) are antisocial and given to sudden destructive rages. They are demanding, envious of others, and overemphasize their own material and physical needs. Out of touch with their own healing powers, they are insensitive to the needs of others.

Basic Story Elements

Myths and stories often resonate with specific internal processes. This reliable pattern invokes well-being and resilience in every cell of your body:

Setting Out: The protagonist sets out in quest of greater love, strength, justice, wisdom, and happiness.

Trouble: One or more obstacles and/or antagonists interfere with the journey.

Help: Wise and benevolent help comes, often giving a gift.

Positive Ending: The protagonist fulfils the quest with joy and celebration.

SUMMONING YOUR STORYTELLER

The thymus personality ensures that everyone's needs are generously and substantially met. They tell stories using words and gestures. They tend to say only what they must say, glad to leave the rest to others. They have a healing and strengthening effect as they induce others through their silent influence to experience physical well-being. They resonate especially with strong silent people to whom they are drawn viscerally. Heroes and heroines with physical charisma transform whatever dark opposing forces interfere with healthy and abundant life.

Exercises to Explore and Balance the Thymus

Songfests and fetes. Nigerian medicine men are said to ask this question: "When is the last time you sang a song or told a story?" What areas of your life could benefit from a celebration? What are you waiting for? Drum up enthusiasm for celebration, like the young man in the story "The Sacred Gift of Celebration." Your house deserves celebration, as much as your body. Purchase a drum or thrum on your chest as you dance and sing.

Take a global step and invoke the well-being of the whole Earth as you celebrate your locality. Plan a community celebration during which everyone will feel abundantly well served. Find a communal space and a good cause. Raise money and spirit that will nourish an underfed population. Purchase a huge communal cooking pot or two and large stirring spoons. Find a celebration drum. Plan dancing, singing, and storytelling—and start the festivities.

Building a house of celebration. Make up a story in which a protagonist and antagonist with the characteristics described meet. End your story with a very positive celebration. Perhaps the wedded pair at the end of a story provide lavish food and entertainment for all their wedding guests. Let all the language in your story refer to physical realities and activities.

Magical table of plenty. Tell a story about a magical table of abundance. For inspiration, read "The Wishing-Table, the Gold-Ass, and the Cudgel in the Sack" in the Grimms' collection of fairy tales. Imagine a traveling master of celebrations who helps people revel in well-being wherever he goes, and tell his story.

Too much abundance. A nanny who was taking care of a modern-day prince described huge palaces and feasts in which her young charge participated. All the royal children in this realm had rooms full of toys and watches and stuffed animals. Everyone was provided for with material opulence beyond reason. Tell a story about children rebelling against material excess to help the whole Earth survive. How do they transform the overabundance with which they have grown up?

Drawing out festivity and jubilation. This color exercise can be repeated again and again to call your body out of the darkness of envy and rage. On a large piece of drawing paper, first express with charcoal or pencil a dark, shadowy underworld. Then transform the shadows with strong vibrant colors that invite the whole world to celebrate generous and jubilant feelings of vitality and healthy abundance with you.

Expanding Thymus Awareness Through Dance, Music, and Yoga

Dance
Beat vigorously or tap on your breastbone and dance, like a king or a queen at the door of a feasting room welcoming your guests.

Music
Berlioz, Overture to *Roman Carnival*
Mouret, Rondeau
Prokofiev, Folk Dance and Masks from *Romeo and Juliet*
Strauss, Waltzes

Yoga asanas (Sanskrit names in italics)
Bridge *(Setu Bandha)*
Shoulder Stand *(Sarvangasana)*
Shoulder Bridge with legs up the wall *(Viparita Karani)*

14

Individualist: The Appendix

Imagine that nothing can destroy you for long, that you have lived for hundreds and thousands of years, and will go on living with ease in new versions of your body. Many tales give voice to this plotline that expresses our most ancient and powerful survival instincts. These tales resonate with the old reptilian mind and body, of which the appendix is a part.

It is not surprising that, like all our organs, which carry on specific functions within us, the appendix hums with its own complex mission. This sensitive drainage area is a sac of power at the bottom of the digestive system. Attached to the entrance of the large intestine at the lower right side of the abdomen, it is a long narrow tube that can heat up and swell from one-half inch to more than three inches in length. Its most well-known task is to deal with overloads of heavy metals and toxins from which the large intestine has been unable to protect itself fully.

Yet your appendix also helps you experience ancient intestinal fortitude; it can bubble at times like a cauldron holding magical ingredients. It is part of an old and powerful immune response system that sometimes leaps suddenly into action within us. Although the appendix is commonly seen as an organ of little importance, many recognize that it is part of the immune system, one of the internal reservoirs that aids recovery from harmful microorganisms and other threats to our survival. Loaded with white blood cells, it is perfectly placed to warn the immune system of invasion. If the appendix detects harm, it heats up to destroy pathogens. It also secretes fluids that lubricate food and stimulate the muscular contractions of the colon that move digestion along. If feces are backed up and toxic, the appendix can plug and swell. Appendicitis is a sign that the appendix is on high alert. If left unattended, as many can attest, it shouts sharp aches and pain on the lower right side, and can even burst and spill its toxic contents into the abdomen.

STIMULATING ESSENTIAL IMMUNE RESPONSE

As he helped himself heal from a bout of appendicitis, Bob Cooley researched the effect of the appendix on the whole body with a group of us in his Meridian Stretching Center through intensive practice of the locust pose. We learned that even when the appendix is removed, it continues to work on a subtle level and can have a sometimes dramatic influence on our whole relationship with life. To begin to experience this primordial energy, massage the path of the large intestine. Focus on the beginning of your ascending colon on your lower right side. Then press and hold your middle and fourth fingers together. In amphibians, these two fingers are often connected as one phalange. Hold these fingers together and lie on your back or side, also pressing your legs firmly together. The effect can be sensational if you contract your lower back and your leg muscles until your back and legs arch upward together. Moving from your lower back, you may find yourself thrashing spontaneously, like a glistening mermaid or merman. Now try lying full-length face down on the floor. As you press your middle and

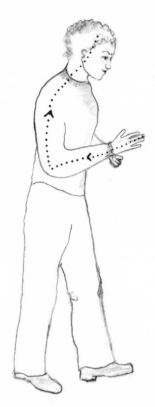

The Appendix "Strange Flow"

fourth fingers together, push down with your palms on the floor. Lift your elbows at either side of your body, like a lizard or alligator. Imagine that your whole torso is lifting up freely behind you. As your elbows press into your sides, energy will move through your palms to your biceps and into your face. You may feel a distinct change of mood as your eyes seem to rotate slightly outward. Place your elbows further under your rib cage so they can carry the weight of your torso. As your legs lift up behind like a tail extension of your backbone, your nose and mouth may push forward slightly, and you will experience for yourself how the appendix connects to the glands deep within the brain.

LEAPING LIZARDS WITHIN

The ancient reptilian-like aspects of our present-day human bodies include not only the appendix, but also the pineal

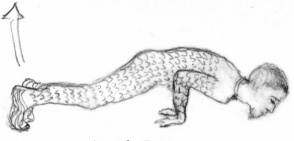

Appendix Exercise

gland, the main gland concerned with sleep and trance. This gland secretes hormones, such as melatonin, that help us to light up from within and to move. Long years of evolution allow us to store and to experience the old sunlight, starlight, and other cosmic formative forces in and around our bodies that sometimes flare up spontaneously from within us, especially in times of stress and need, to reveal a way forward.

The pineal gland is part of a sensing eye that once dominated the middle of the forehead. This old hidden "third eye" has gradually receded, yet sometimes still releases ancient powers of clairvoyance in both children and adults. Clairvoyance gives us the ability to see spontaneously beyond our immediate world of time and space. Most of us today rarely have visions of events and places that do not occur in our immediate surroundings. Yet some people are able to open inner seeing at will, and without depending on rational perception or study, see into past and future times and places, and there meet past and future lives. This also gives us a sense of our potential for sudden evolutionary changes.

Traditional Chinese medicine refers to "strange flows" that do not follow specific pathways and seem to be still older than meridians; in outlandish ways these can deeply influence the whole body. Bob Cooley's experimental work with this appendix area woke me up to this "strange flow" in my own body. As I was experimenting with the formative and protective energy related to the old reptilian body through yoga exercises and I began to contact this part of myself, my whole body would gather into stillness, as if trying to become invisible. Then it would suddenly leap forward with lizard-like ease and power. I noticed that my tongue would become very active. I also became more light sensitive than usual. Colors would fade, and instead I saw light and shadows playing through the bodies of my friends. I began to have a vivid sense of how reptilian limbs, unlike our human limbs, can regenerate themselves.

Snakes and lizards not only have the ability to restore limbs, they can also change their colors and molt their skins, as some sea creatures cast off their shells. Many can scurry back and forth between water and land, more open to extraterrestrial sensations because they are not yet exclusively Earth beings. The chilly vestigial reptilian network within us intermeshes with our warmer mammalian life body to give us subtle awareness of profound cyclic changes. It puts us in touch with our most powerful impulses for molting and transformation, both long, slow, undulating changes and rapturous moments of purging and leaping forward into new life.

A primal sense of vigilance illuminates people who live strongly with the powerful old survival powers that are concentrated in the old reptilian brain and body. They tend to live apart, as if they are perpetual newcomers from an alien world. From a watchful distance, they avoid the turmoil of earthly events and emotions. Sensing that they might be misunderstood or disregarded, they may sit, as if on a rock, awaiting ultimate illuminations, and let the world pass by. Their leapfrogging activities might include bungee jumping and hang gliding. Their inner lives and their social lives tend to be unusual. They are most content when they can create professional lives that allow them to live in the energy of sudden leaps. They read swiftly changing trends. As businesspeople, they can "see" and target markets far into the future. Sometimes they become professional psychics who are able to see into past and future events. Often interested in science fiction, they tend to feel mysteriously in touch with influences beyond this earthly one, yet long to feel more ordinary and less extraterrestrial. Like Saint-Exupéry's prince in his masterpiece *Le Petit Prince,* they tend to make others feel like strangers on Earth, too. Some harness higher spiritual powers as seers, oracles, and prophets to change the world. Isaiah's voice rings through the ages. Saint John warns: "The light shineth in the darkness and the darkness comprehendeth it not." John the Baptist cries in the wilderness to prepare the way for utmost spiritual truth.

Many who are especially in touch with the ancient reptilian energy body need much privacy and may seem to disappear or take on protective coloration to disguise the intensity of their inner lives. "I don't connect with people very well," explained one of these folks. "As a child I had little to say. I was working on my own level. People misunderstand me all the time. I am not quick to respond to others because I am thinking and sensing. I can't connect right away. I live on the peripheries and I don't belong to any group. I am just here on Earth riding *maya.*"

A man who lives strongly in this realm needed to better define his highly sensitive individuality. He decided to divorce his wife in order to go on actually living with her and their children. For relief from the strain of their domestic life, he regularly retreats to his sailboat to hover in his favorite comfort zone between sea and land. A skillful anesthetist, he monitors patients as they go into limbo and return changed. He, too, says he is slow to connect with his emotions. "I can administer anesthesia fearlessly. When there is trouble, I am innately wired so I don't panic," he explains, "but this doesn't serve well in intimate relationships. I take a long while to sort out my feelings and I take a very distant view to protect myself."

Indeed, life can feel like a dream journey as this old energetic system, in connection with the pineal and pituitary glands, activates threshold experiences beyond the ordinary bounds of time and space. Contemporary astrophysics suggests that we live in an endlessly transforming universe without fixed beginning or end. Astronomers and other scientists increasingly acknowledge our kinship with the solar system and countless wheeling galaxies beyond, as they attempt through scientific means to establish communication with other worlds beyond Earth. Such physicists quip: "The surest sign that there are other intelligences in this universe is that they have made no attempt to contact ours."

When appendix and old reptilian brain activity predominates, it can lead to highly unusual personalities. When I lived in England, I befriended a professional healer who lived intensely on the border between life and death. He had healed himself of many illnesses and so was able to help others. Being curious and eager, I wanted to learn from him, but soon discovered how individual his methods were. He worked alone and had little connection with his own emotions or feelings, except as they served his work. He went barefoot even in winter. Though he was married, he had no children. His wife went her own way as an artist, and he kept close watch over her health. He seemed always prepared to bring about intensive healing to those desperate enough to call in his aid. He loved to drive his car at very high speeds; the local police had learned to leave him alone, as he moved so adeptly and did no harm. Through a special apparatus that he was ever perfecting, he was able to tap into his patients' precise imbalances to facilitate their healing, whether physical, emotional, mental, or spiritual. Largely self-trained in medical diagnostics, he had mastered much knowledge of the vibratory fields of illnesses. He lived "under his rock" in a small English village until a call came to him for help. Then he would spring to action. He ate little food, had a wild sense of humor, and generally found human life extremely strange. Although at that time I had given little thought to the possibility of reincarnation, I had the distinct impression that he was correcting for a previous lifetime of great destructiveness, perhaps as a soldier who had killed with terrible skill hundreds or perhaps thousands of other souls.

Those who evolve in this realm and serve others can do great good. Another uniquely effective, cranky, and hilarious healer from whom I tried to learn referred to his patients as "humanoids." He, too, had discovered and crossed over thresholds that most people gladly avoid. He lived largely on a diet of elm bark, avocadoes, and alfalfa, and when he was not busy writing a huge science fiction saga to change the world, he supported his quick, slender, shamanic body, and also his elderly parents, by giving his eccentric, holistic health consultations. Quick to recognize false or whiney excuses, he had eerie insight into where the shadows fell on people's spirits and overall health. He usually offered brusque guidance for comprehensive transformation to a much simpler and healthier lifestyle.

In such people, apocalyptic light filters into the earthier mammalian nervous system. In extreme instances, the intensity of this light can sometimes strike a person temporarily dumb and blind. Loss of speech altogether can result in instant insight, a new openness to light and vision beyond the ordinary. Though the outer eye may be blind and the speech struck dumb, a higher sensing may awaken to ignite speaking that seems to come from other realms. A new kind of listening, too, may bring surprising guidance and a catapulting in a new direction.

The Book of Jonah in the Old Testament shows that being a messenger for God to instigate transformations is not necessarily an easy role. Jonah preferred to hide from his prophetic calling, but the God force in his spirit compelled him to go where he was sent to warn people to change their ways. Even when his boat foundered in a storm, there was no turning back. He was destined to move out of the water to instigate evolution. Swallowed by a mysterious fish, Jonah was held safely for three days and three nights in its watery belly, then spewed onto a shore nearer his destination.

Ego and Individuality: The Sense of Self

Change is a constant theme in every human life; sacred spirit within us attracts these changes. In *Alice's Adventures in Wonderland,* Lewis Carroll wrote:

"Who are you?" said the Caterpillar. "I—I hardly know, Sir, just at present," Alice replied rather shyly. "At least I know who I was when I got up this morning, but I think I must have changed several times since then."

According to Rudolf Steiner, the body's ability to hold and transform poisons has helped us evolve sufficient antipathy for maintaining a sense of personal identity. The stinging, even fatal poisons that snakes and other cold-blooded reptiles use to defend themselves transformed gradually into the ego forces in human beings. The human ego becomes part of everyone's unique immune defense system. As inner selfhood develops in connection with the internal immune system, it acquires some of the intractable powers of a lizard on a rock.

"The Six Swans" in the Grimms' collection, and in the Irish myth "The Children of Lir," portray young people as especially sensitive to the stinging powers of self-transformation. As they build themselves up from within, they need much protection. When I was a young teacher, I often shared mythology and poetry with troubled children who lived in abusive circumstances. I wanted them to know the Greek myth of Daphne, the daughter of the river god Peneus, who transformed into a tree for protection against the lust of Apollo. Writing in a Greek persona helped them too feel their way into the story and to express their feelings. I asked them to begin their writing assignment with: "Long and far and young ago, when I was a warrior in the land called Peloponnesus, I heard this told." To find my own relationship with this myth, I wrote my own version, in which a maiden bent over a streamlet in the shade of a laurel grove:

The drinking water was sweet there.
The urn she submerged in the gurgling waters
wavered strangely with mosses and minnows.
She smelt her own cleanliness as she felt the brook's dancing coolness.
She lifted her hem to wade deep in its kindness.

Suddenly, Apollo burst beating his lust toward her beauty.
She flailed her arms and her breath failed.
In vain did she call to her father, her mother.
Ugly and trembling, she was a rabbit to his joy.
She groaned, gathering her wholeness.
"O Father," was her plea, "to a place beyond hiding let me go. Let me be."

Then the Mother of Mercy heard her pleading
"Bequeath your feet to me.
I shall root you truly. Hold fast."

The terrified Daphne, when these words were spoken,
stepped outward with dignity onto a treeless field.
The goddess breathed her protection.
Changing, she grew less, yet was safe now.
Though her heart trembled into branches,
and her feet swelled, delving the earth,
she who was skittish in darkness of fear
now turned into brightness and budding.

She was tree now, of the one Tree—
She sings. Time holds her.
Flown into the heart of a greater Light,
Apollo sends gentle birds into her arms.

THE VICTORIOUS MONKEY KING

Heroes and heroines with maverick powers of transformation abound in many cultures. Children growing up in China often hear about a magical monkey king. It is said that this fabulous monkey trickster was deposited in the form of a stone egg on a mountain during a huge storm.

A dragon breathed fire on this egg. The egg burned for nine days and nights. On the tenth day, in place of the stone egg, stood a small stone monkey. The next day a gentle breeze tickled the monkey and his eyes opened. Rain turned his stone skin into silky golden fur. He wriggled his fingers and toes, flexed his muscles, and laughed a long mischievous laugh. His eyes shone with strange light.

Born so mysteriously between heaven and earth, this little monkey was immediately able to leap great distances. One day he leapt fearlessly into a waterfall. Beneath the waterfall, he found a paradise garden. Other monkeys, admiring his bursting independent will, joined him there and made him their king. But soon this renegade monkey could not resist setting out in search of the secrets of eternal life. He found a teacher of the path to immortality. A wildly maverick student, at last he returned to his monkey people when they were captured by a "demon of havoc," a destructive force that had come upon them like a tornado, filling the sky with darkness and roaring.

"Don't worry," said the monkey to the other monkeys. "I'll get him." He sprang high into the sky. His penetrating vision searched over thousands of miles until he saw a dark swirling mist on a faraway mountain. Riding on a cloud, Monkey darted off and landed next to a vast hole with stinking toxic fumes rolling out of it.

"Who dares to challenge me?" screamed a poisonous voice, and the next moment the havoc leapt out of the hole. He was enormous. His eyes were fireballs. In each hand he carried lightning bolts.

Monkey made himself invisible. "Here I am! Here I am!" he taunted, leaping here, there, and everywhere.

The demon struck madly, but each time he struck nothing but air. Finally, the demon began to tire. Then Monkey paused to pluck several golden hairs from his own leg. These turned immediately into hundreds of tiny monkeys that swarmed all over the demon— pulling, kicking, even tickling him. They knocked him down so that he couldn't get up again. Monkey then reappeared in his natural form and leapt into the demon's stinking poisonous lair. He plunged downward until he found his monkey friends tied together, like trapped crabs.

"Hurry," cried the monkey, "we're going home!" The demon was afraid to move. "Never hurt my clan again!" the monkey warned, "or it will be even worse for you." From there he flew home with all his monkey friends holding onto his tail.

Monkey organized the other monkeys into a mighty and powerful nation.

"No one will be able to defeat us again. No one!" claimed the monkey.

THE ALCHEMY OF EVOLUTION

The monkey king's seemingly magical leaping lizard power resembles the internal immune system when it has been activated by an emergency, and his organizing of the other monkeys the intricate and cooperative nature of this system. Every individual must cultivate survival tactics throughout the long evolutionary drama of the human body and soul over many lifetimes. An individual soul can gradually evolve toward saintly wisdom and complete enlightenment. The Old Testament prophet Isaiah envisioned sudden transformations of all humanity and the Earth. Rumi's spiritual teacher arrived like a bolt of lightning and changed Rumi's entire life. Stories of Nasrudin in the Arabic world and of the Baal Shem Tov in Jewish culture attest to the immense potential of swift self-transformation within individuals whose inner core is strong and who, like "Jumping Mouse" in the American Indian tale, are willing to endure the joy and pain of transformation.

Buddhists recount the lives of the Buddha and his evolutionary journey through countless life forms, deaths, and rebirths as he built up a fully integrated body of spiritual wisdom. Many of the episodes that led to the complete enlightenment of the Buddha survive in the *jataka* texts that are said to be at least twenty-five hundred years old. Rafe Martin's *The Hungry Tigress* contains a fine selection of these tales, together with his inspiring commentaries.

Antoine de Saint-Exupéry piloted mail through night skies for many months as he dreamt of his book *Le Petit Prince*. The hero of this book is a resilient extraterrestrial who is learning to love. Much science fiction is written in a similar mood, from outside and above, with heroes and heroines who ignore the laws of ordinary space and time and possess strange powers.

The Necessary Poetry of Transformation

Taliesen, a legendary Welsh hero born in the days of Arthur, came to life because of a woman of great power, named Ceridwen (pronounced Ker'-id-wen). Her beloved son was so ugly that she wanted him to excel in other ways.

◦❦◦❦◦❦◦

The Cauldron of Ceridwen

Ceridwen consulted her books of knowledge until she found in an old book a spell for the Cauldron of Inspiration. The recipe called for wheat, honey, incense, myrrh, aloes, silver, and fluxwort. These she mixed with the red berries sometimes called rowan. And she stirred in cress and vervain, plucked when the Dog Star was rising. She set this cauldron to simmer as the book directed, for one year and one day exactly.

She ordered her servant, Gwion Bach, to stir it slowly and keep it at a gentle bubble. This he did all day every day, until one morning near the end of the appointed time, three drops splashed onto his finger. Cooling his scalded finger in his mouth, the young lad knew at once the past, the present, and the future. He had received what Ceridwen had intended for her son, and so he rushed forth as the cauldron cracked into one thousand pieces. All that remained was deadly poison.

When Ceridwen heard the cauldron crack, she chased her servant, but Gwion Bach became a hare. She became a hound and ran hot on his heels. He became a fish to foil the hound. She became an otter and nearly snatched him. He became a dove to foil the otter. She became a hawk who, with huge flaps of her wings, was about to overtake the exhausted dove. As his strength failed, he became a groat in a pile of wheat. But she became a black hen, and scuffed at the wheat until she found the one grain that was Gwion Bach. She pecked him up, and swallowed him whole.

But that was not the end of Gwion Bach. In the course of time, Ceridwen gave birth to another son who was Gwion. She bound this son in a bag of skins and cast him into the sea. The bag went with the waves until the passing of King Arthur into the time of King Maelgwn, a long time indeed, and at last the bag was caught in salmon nets near Aberystwyth. Every May, the king there granted salmon rights to whom he favored, and that year it was to his own son, Elfin. This lad, a wastrel, waded out to where the long nets were staked across the river mouth and hauled the bag ashore, thinking he might find jewels in it. But instead, out leapt the baby from the mouth of the bag, speaking words of power and music and wisdom that may never have been heard before by any human ears. Fresh from the alchemical bag, the light that streamed from the babe's face was so bright that Elfin named him Taliesen, which means Shining Brow.

Said Elfin to his father, "I caught a Poet." The old king bemoaned all this strangeness, and it was then that Taliesen spoke his first words:

I am Taliesen
I sing perfect meter which will last till the world's end.
I have been a blue salmon,
a dog, a stag, a roebuck on the mountain, a stock, a spade, an axe in the hand,
a buck, a bull, a stallion upon a hill. I was grown as grain,
reaped, and in the oven thrown.
Out of that roasting I fell to the ground,
pecked up and swallowed by a black hen. In her crop nine nights lain.
I have been dead. I have been alive.
I am Taliesen.

⌘⌘⌘⌘⌘

TRANSFORMING COLD ENVY

When powers of self-transformation are cramped, they can turn cruel. The dark underbelly of the survival skills held in the appendix is cold-blooded, detached. Within everyone is a cold, envious pit of snakes that feed on warm-blooded life—a public relations expert in reverse who refuses warmth, attachment, and loving support. Here stories from many lands depict strange semi-human entities whose adaptive powers are oddly toxic. Like Golem in *The Lord of the Rings,* they may have elongated pointer fingers and toes, bumpy toadlike facial skin, and large gleaming eyes.

"The Crystal Ball" in the Grimm collection portrays a misshapen enchantress who has three sons. She envies their manliness and fears that they will steal her power from her. With sly, cold magic, she changes the eldest into an eagle, which is forced to fly in great circles in the sky. The second she changes into a whale, which lives in the deep sea. The third, rather than be turned into a wild beast, goes secretly away and develops his own powers of transformation. With a magic wishing cap, he enters the Castle of the Golden Sun and disenchants the beautiful princess who has been captured there. Then he frees his brothers from their captivity. Together they also liberate the sublime Crystal Ball of Truth that their mother had hidden away in the castle.

TRANSFORMATIONAL STORYTELLING

Appendix Affirmation

I transform to become enlightened.

Basic Appendix Story Dynamic

Aloneness turns into prophetic wisdom.

Appendix Protagonists and Antagonists

Appendix protagonists (characters who support appendix health) are assertive, energetic, and deeply intuitive. They are adaptable individualists who are aware of past and future lives and extraterrestrial, futuristic phenomena. They bring about sudden changes of consciousness.

Appendix antagonists (characters who express appendix dysfunction) stifle individualism. They are morbid anarchists, crusading, disapproving, and destructive. They leap ahead in thought and deed without concern for others.

Basic Story Elements

Myths and stories often resonate with specific internal processes. This reliable pattern invokes well-being and resilience in every cell of your body:

Setting Out: The protagonist sets out in quest of greater love, strength, justice, wisdom, and happiness.

Trouble: One or more obstacles and/or antagonists interfere with the journey.

Help: Wise and benevolent help comes, often giving a gift.

Positive Ending: The protagonist fulfils the quest with joy and celebration.

SUMMONING YOUR STORYTELLER

The ancient consciousness of these storytellers is capable of leaping with lightning speed into the future. They bring science fiction to life. Extraordinarily light sensitive, they possess primal intuitive powers that draw on humans' deepest survival instincts and evolutionary powers. The story worlds they inhabit are full of danger and magical transformations. They have a tendency to contract and crouch, ready to spring forward with intense gestures and the darting speed of a lizard's tongue. Eyes narrow, on hyper alert, with wide peripheral vision, their sight is directed beyond conventional reality to include the extraterrestrial. Their garments provide them with chameleon-like protection, as with cool detachment they sense whether others are friend or foe.

Exercises to Explore and Balance the Realm of the Appendix

Merlin's accomplice. With our subtle bodies, we can clothe ourselves in any shape we choose. Imagine a character in a story, like young King Arthur when he was in training with Merlin, the great wizard and enchanter. In Celtic tradition, Arthur's preparation for his kingly duties is incomplete until he fully experiences the real lives of rocks, plants, and animals, and learns how to pass successfully through those realms. Choose one of the natural realms and imagine yourself inhabiting that realm for a time. Give your poetic voice a fling. Describe your experiences, for example, as a fish, or a blade of grass, or a prehistoric snake. Be sure to include lessons learned in each realm.

Dowsing light and shadow. Sit as still as a lizard on a rock and observe the play of light and shadow on objects and around people. Try to sense the light and dark in the people's thoughts and feelings.

Into the fire. Imagine you have lived for thousands of years and that you will go on living. Look at the world through those eyes. Nothing can destroy you for long. Describe your life three hundred years or light years from now. Take an evolutionary plunge forward. Surrender yourself to the wisest possible human evolution. Imagine six swift transformations you would choose to undergo in order to develop yourself more fully. List these. Then take some time to picture your fears and doubts as a variety of creatures that are pursuing and stimulating you to keep moving ahead until you have changed your ways. Write this as a whole story and then speak your story aloud, as you crouch ready to spring forward into a new life, perhaps bringing many others along with you.

Cast a spell. We all live under various spells for a time. A haiku by the Japanese poet Basho reads:

In my new robe
This morning
Someone else.

Playfully break out of an old fixation. Molt the past. Give yourself a new identity, a different bodily shape with a new set of goals. Go in search of a new outfit to help you inhabit this new reality.

EXPANDING APPENDIX AWARENESS THROUGH DANCE, MUSIC, AND YOGA

Dance

With your tongue extended and pressing your two middle fingers together as if they are one, crouch like a lizard under a safe rock, studying the light. Hide in shadow, and then leap suddenly forward, as if you can see your distant goal through a far-scanning eye in the middle of your forehead. Continue your dance in this mood, sometimes moving with your whole body on the floor, as if you are lighting your way forward by a beam of light projected from the middle of your forehead. Keep your elbows bent, strong and fluid, and your tongue moving back and forth like an extra hand sensing your environment to help you find the way forward.

Music
Holst, *The Planets*
Stravinsky, The Evocation of the Ancestors and Sacrificial Dance from *Le Sacre du Printemps*
Hindemith, *Viola Concerto*
Shostakovich, *Symphony in Three Movements,* the first movement

Yoga asanas (Sanskrit names in italics)
Locust *(Salabhasana, Poorna-Salabhasana)*
Peacock *(Mayurasana)*
Frog *(Mandukasana)*

15

Voluptuary: The Genitals

"Every human being is the universe kissing the earth," says Brother Blue, who is often called the grandfather of American storytelling. The body's keen old moderators for our many erogenous zones work diligently to regulate the vast magnetic forces from which we are made. As both cosmic and earthly energies form our bodies for love from dazzling polarities, we are inevitably attractive. Whether you are madly and magnificently mating, or have temporarily fallen out of love and would like to feel irresistible, to invite wild and wonderful feelings, breathe into your belly. Let your chest and neck relax. Now press your elbows against your ribs, making small rhythmic circles with them while keeping them pressed against the sides of your body. Move slowly to wake up subtle muscles by arching your torso as you contract your back muscles and stretch the whole front of your body. As your head falls back, keep your elbows close to your body and contract all the muscles of your lower back. Beautiful energy will rise from your legs through your belly to your chin, and blossom through your lips. As you breathe more deeply, wink flirtatiously and let a primal and playful chant of desire sound from deep within you.

For a more intensive experience, sit on the floor with your legs stretched straight out before you and tighten your belly. Now lift your feet a little at a time, and breathe into your belly until sexual energies spring forth willy-nilly with a life all their own—projecting and asserting, receiving and embracing.

Life desires itself with wild persistence. The meridians that relate directly to sexuality prove that generative passion is truly a full-bodied affair. The Conception Vessel, as it is called in

Chinese medicine, originates in the pelvis, dips slightly between the anus and genitalia, then ascends through the torso to the root of the tongue. From there, it encircles the lips and branches to the eyes.

Sexual energies love to circulate with passionate determination in both body and soul, closing gaps wherever they can. Unbounded in their mission, these strategic regenerative unifying forces strive to bring us all into intimate relationships, causing us to preen and groom our fine points, and respond to one another as to a magnet. As life powers are gathered together, so an entirely new organism has the possibility of coming into being via our reproductive organs. With sublime innocence, the unbounded true lover within us inspires only confidence in life and love. A feisty Scots storyteller who sports a kilt is often asked what he wears underneath it. "Nothing is worrrn," he says with his characteristic candor and poise, "and everything is in perrrrrfect working order."

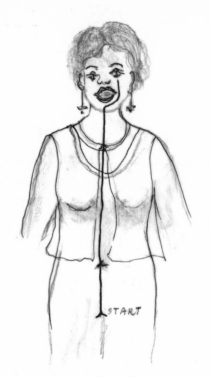

The Conception Vessel

BEING AS WONDERFUL AS YOU ARE

Like Maya Angelou and Walt Whitman, many long to express in poetry and song the concentrated flux of emotions that belong to orgasmic vitality. Revelers who live the life of desire seem always to be in a courting mood. They feel with infinitely generous self-absorption: "I am the one, the center-pin. Why would you want anyone else?" To the question "Do you feel attractive?" lovers reply without hesitation, "Of course." Although they may wonder briefly if their clothes are a little awkward or whether they have spinach on their front teeth, riding irresistible waves of delectable hormones, inciting flirtations in a moment, they feel loveable to their very toes.

An eighty-year-old friend says with orgasmic elegance and the authority of a goddess, "I love attracting others to glorious events. I have created and attended so many through the years! I feel everyone, young and old, should be celebrated as much as possible. Birthdays should have a big momentum. I let everyone know about mine in advance. My husband and I always invite friends and carolers to join us in a fabulous feast in the evening, to serenade us with violins, woodwinds, and brass." When I ask, "How did you get to be this way, the unabashed center of attraction?" she answers simply, "I always thank everyone and everything that makes me as wonderful as I am."

Voluptuous personalities include many helpful male and female receptionists, models and couturiers, nurses, socialites, salespeople, hairdressers, and endearing waiters and waitresses.

When we meet these solicitous people, we feel drawn to being taken care of by them. We may want to shout, "Hey, wait a minute! Is this seduction? How am I going to get out of this?" Or perhaps we think to ourselves, "Maybe I don't want to get out of this at all."

"I love hearing what you're saying" is the impression a school receptionist gives to all children, parents, and visitors. For her second job, she sings and waits tables. She responds to others' needs sometimes before they are even aware of them. She gives the feeling that each person is exciting, wonderful, and important. "You belong right here with me," she seems to be saying. With exultant focus, she puts cup with saucer. With unabashed décolletage, she is available, flushed, excited, and joyous. In response to the intensity of her feelings, she teases her hair until it stands on end.

Courtesans and gigolos, models and crooning stars of stage and screen, promotional experts—all the magnetic sexual personalities throughout the world inhabit an ancient place to which everyone is coming. Stars of stage and screen exude this energy. As they come to believe more fully in themselves and what they can do, as they move into the spotlight, their sense of being irresistible can intensify. Only a hardened cynic can resist their power, as they soften all our parts, support comfort, and ignite love and beauty. They start dating agencies. They love to hear us disclose the most intimate secrets of our lives.

THE EXCITEMENT OF BEING IN DEEP TROUBLE

The whole history of sexuality lives in our bodies, and gives rise to personality quirks and endless stories. A much loved nurse often cut loose from her responsibilities to go on passionate adventures, lurching about in colorful vehicles that she bought on credit and just as impulsively traded in for the next one. She explains, "For years nothing others said made a difference to my behavior. During these wild bouts, my emotions had a life of their own; too often they would govern me. I went against police and judges because I didn't want to follow rules. I was recognized about town as a chaotic belligerent 'bitch,' getting attention in the wrong way. But now," she insists, "I take care of my business. I have learned to go deeper within myself. I have been a slow learner because I had to experience my emotions for myself from within my own body."

STORIES THAT STIMULATE HEALTHY SEXUALITY

Desire can feel chaotic and cause much trouble, yet its magic also creates balance and joy as, with infinite orgasmic ingenuity, it gathers and submits us to its power. The great magic of fertility will endure until the last child is born on Earth. We are wondrously made through a vastly ardent process in which we must participate. New human beings ever long to dive into the womb and to be assembled mysteriously by illuminated hands that have mastered minute instructions.

Some cultures shy away from matters that are sexually explicit; others celebrate this aspect of our humanity with tremendous verve. Chaucer, Shakespeare, Boccaccio, and Rumi are all masters of this realm, their stories and poems often acting as teachers and guides for sexual development.

In the North American Indian tradition, trickster Coyote sees a beautiful woman and sends his penis across wide water to make love with her. A watchful elder straddles it and drives a spike through it. Coyote's passion abruptly cools for a time. A wise and playful storyteller from the Limba people of northern Sierra Leone tells of the origin of our sexual parts.

The Creation of the Sexes

May my tale give you joy! Once long ago, in the beginning, not long after this world was brought out, Kanu Masala brought forth into the light the first person: an old woman. At first, Old Woman, she was happy to be alive! Looking around at this beautiful world, feeling the sun on her skin, tasting all the fruits, she let the juice run down her chin. But after a while, she got to wondering what her purpose was on this earth. So she went back to Kanu Masala and said, "Kanu, since you have brought me into the light of day, then tell me, what am I to do here?"

"All right," said Kanu. "I will give you some work to do." So Kanu Masala went off and stood and thought, and by and by, he made a man, for there was no man here on earth at all. And then he made a woman, this time a beautiful young woman. And then Kanu brought a basket to Old Woman. "Old Woman, these are for you to sell."

Old Woman looked at what Kanu had brought her. "What's all this?"

"This is your merchandise. People will be coming along soon and when they do, you can sell this to them."

Old Woman looked at Kanu and then back at the merchandise. "People will want this?"

"Oh yes, very much! Women need two of these and one of those. Men need one of those and two of these."

"Really?"

Kanu nodded.

So Old Woman, she started sorting out and hanging up the merchandise as Kanu began to walk away, but then she thought of another question. "Kanu, where do they keep them?"

Kanu walked back over, looked around, and when he was sure that they were alone, he whispered in Old Woman's ear.

"Really?" she asked.

Kanu smiled and nodded.

"No!"

"Really!" Kanu grinned.

"But don't they get in the way?"

Kanu shook his head.

"But what do people *do* with this merchandise? How does it work?"

"Trust me, Old Woman. You just tell the people to put these things together, and everything will come out all right."

And with that said, Kanu went along on his way.

༺༻

GETTING TO YES

Learning to live with sexual parts and sexual impulses begins early in childhood. Betty Peck, an educator of young children for more than fifty years, placed the letters of the alphabet in golden wooden cutouts as high as they would go on the wall of her kindergarten room, interspersed among stars. When she brought down a letter to teach it to the children, it was always a grand event. She and the children celebrated each letter of the alphabet, dancing and singing words and eating foods in honor of each. When the children discovered the one complete word in the very middle of the whole sequence of the alphabet—NO—Mrs. Peck helped them to play with it in many ways through story, rhyme, and song until they could all say it in many moods.

Eventually came the story of a king who ruled with his queen in justice and love. "I am a good ruler," spoke the king. "I know the rules!" he said. "The queen and I stand in the middle of the realm and we say, "No, no one in school touches your private parts. Private means private." Mrs. Peck pointed to the letters as she said each "no." And that was that. No discussion. No waffling. Just setting the rules in her classroom realm. Formidable Mrs. Peck didn't name the parts scientifically. She simply called them "private parts," and got on with teaching the children about reproduction by observing the lives of plants and of animals. This teacher also sent clear messages to parents about the rules of the realm in school. Mrs. Peck never had an incident of children acting out inappropriate sexuality in her classroom. She created what she wanted, a safe place for children, and for their parents, too.

Sexuality teaches us to ride its tidal rhythms in body and soul as daily we give birth to more of who we are. Who is easy with sexuality for long without challenge? When I was a young woman, I found myself overwhelmed by my own fertility, and also by the growing magnitude of the world's population. The children that my lovers and I might have together visited me in dreams; I would sometimes see rivers of babies coming to the shore of the earth. One bright spring day, striding in Manhattan and feeling the fecundity within me, I looked up. Towering on both sides were tall apartment buildings, their windows gleaming with white light. At that moment, the sense of so many multitudes of people living on top of one another in cities all over the world—their courtships, couplings, marriage beds, molestations, rapes—every imaginable sexual expression gathered to one point within me. A measureless compassion opened up within me, for myself, and for everyone as sexual beings. I resolved to master these rampant and chaotic sexual forces, and to learn to help others to transform them, too.

Many years later, when I began to practice psychotherapy, I rented a house in the country with a beautiful open hearth. There I met with people who wanted to heal areas of their lives that were blocked from happiness and expression. A woman arrived to explore a very painful theme in her childhood: her seven-year sexual relationship with her older brother.

She had managed to forget it in the richness of her marriage and life with her own growing children. But now she was restless and wanted to explore the feelings of rage and sorrow that were surfacing again in order to transform them. I asked why her successful middle-class American parents had provided no rituals to protect them from their incestuous relationship. What was happening between her mother and father that they forgot to remember their children's need for sexual guidance?

It was a dim overcast morning. The hearth fire sparkled. I brought out clay and she took a moist handful from the container and formed it into a phallus. "It is young," she said, "adolescent." She pounded the clay erection that had formed between her hands repeatedly against the hearth-stone. Then she threw the cold little phallus away. She lay down on her back and screamed. After a while, she sat up and looked sorrowfully at me. She moaned. Then she was shouting, "I hate him. I hate him!" I felt moved to get my American Indian ceremonial turtle rattle and my tambourine. I shook them tentatively to echo her words and feelings. After a while, she screamed out, "I want to kill him!" So I gripped harder on the dried leathery turtle neck that was forever extended from the old shell of the Seneca Indian rattle. At that moment, like a bleak, ancient erection, it filled my right hand. I pounded the edge of the shell on the taut round skin of the tambourine. I moved around her as she lay screaming. We had gone quite suddenly to a primal level. This was unexpected for her and for me. We were being drawn into an elemental ritual together.

A cleansing had begun. Like a dancing shaman in this surprising ritual, I remembered, in a flash, a dream that had awakened me the previous year, just before spring. In this dream, a woman lay on her back in the dawn. Behind her a large circle was suspended on a frame, on which an animal skin was stretched taut. The frame was covered with symbolic designs. From a distance there came toward her a powerful male dancer. Both woman and man knew their task. The man was naked except for a headdress and a huge leather penis fastened to his hips that extended out before him. The tribal penis was decorated for this dance with marvelous symbols. Small objects were suspended from it, each with meaning, and he was dancing the penis for everyone and everything. The woman lay expectant before him at a particular distance, energetically correct for the power of the dance. At his approach, the energy gathered between them. The dance required supernatural strength, enough to kill. The couple held all the potency of life between them. Like the early season of spring, they had the power to hold off the orgasm and to gather its strength for the sake of the land and the whole tribe, to bring all the old to a new beginning.

Remembering this dream helped me to follow the healing imagination that unfolded for the troubled woman who sat by the fire. Phantoms of the woman's child self at age seven, at ten, at thirteen appeared to her. Suddenly, she reached for a wooden pointer from the dry kindling at the side of the hearth. From the fire she lit the end of the wand-like stick and moved it like a blessing. It was cleansing her hair, her neck, her breasts, her legs, her hands. Inside and out it was cleansing her.

After a while she came to herself in a new way, saying with the peaceful authority she had never heard from her elders, "Sex is a fiery ocean in which we all live. I bless you. We bless one another. Brothers and sisters grow up and love each other more through their spouses and children. When you are old enough, you will choose well, and mate wisely and respectfully. Brothers and sisters in the same families must choose not to have sex with one another. This is an ancient law. It is like breathing. Everyone must obey. The great pleasure of sex and having children must wait. Later you will know complete love and marriage. You will be glad for one another's happiness." Afterward she found deeply inspired words to resolve within her the story that had troubled her. Her brother, then a well-known lawyer, agreed to listen to her as never before. Eventually, they faced together the effects of their actions, and he offered her a completely heartfelt apology.

COSMIC GODS AND GODDESSES OF DESIRE

Creation stories are among the most sacred in all healthy cultures, where private sexuality is attuned to cosmic creative power. Jan Blake, a radiant, sensuous role model for many other storytellers, often tells this sacred story of the Yoruba people of Nigeria and their descendants, the Orisha who inhabit islands in the Caribbean.

The Loveliest of Women

Once there was a beautiful woman by the name of Ye-ma-ya who looked into the waters of the ocean. There she saw her own reflection and she asked, "Who is that beautiful woman? I thought that I was the prettiest that the world had ever seen!"

And as she looked on that woman there came a rumbling in her belly and it grew and it grew and it grew—until it exploded, and covered the land with lakes, rivers, and streams. Ye-ma-ya looked into the river and again she saw her own reflection and asked, "Who is that beautiful woman?" And again her belly grew and it grew and it grew and it grew—until it exploded, and sprinkled the heavens with stars and a full moon. Ye-ma-ya looked at the full moon, and again she asked, "Who is that beautiful woman? I thought I was the prettiest the world had ever seen." And again her belly grew. And it grew and it grew—until it exploded. And before her stood countless beautiful women. Ye-ma-ya asked, "Who are you, beautiful women? I thought that I was the prettiest the world had ever seen."

The women looked deep into the eyes of Ye-ma-ya and there they saw their own reflections.

So the women said to her, "You are Ye-ma-ya! We are all of you!"

⋯⋯⋯⋯

COSMIC ROMANCE

The storytelling self holds both masculine and feminine in a luminous core of wholeness. We may all appear at times to be in strong union with the ultimate unity and creative force behind gender. As the full cosmic magnitude of sexual feelings are aroused, especially those who most inhabit the sexual realm can give an impression that they are the embodiment of real gods and goddesses. Our earthly sexual saga may lift at times to join with the beauty and luminosity of the night sky as the Milky Way, like mother's milk and perpetual starry seminal fluid, streams across the dark coverlet of space.

Stories give us hints of ancient sexual secrets evolved through long eons of cosmic time. This long evolutionary saga of our human sexuality can be seen glimmering even within babies and the very old. This myth from ancient India pictures a very old sacred drama of sexual union and power.

⋯⋯⋯⋯

Churning the Milky Ocean

The gods and the demons were growing old. They had a common desire to live eternally, without disease, old age, or death. They knew that they must seek the elixir of immortality. This could only be achieved by the churning of the celestial milky ocean. Both gods and demons joined together in this task. They turned the holy mountain Meru upside down for their churning stick. Next they took hold of the sacred body of the snake Vasugi and twined it around the base of the uprooted mountain. As the gods pulled on the snake rope from one side, the demons pulled from the other. From the churning arose a poison strong enough to destroy the world. Fortunately, Shiva took the poison into his mouth and held it in his throat.

Then arose a white elephant, a horse with wings, a wish-fulfilling cow, and many other wonders. Lastly came a great sage bearing the elixir of immortality. The demons immediately snatched this from him. They were about to drink it when Vishnu decided to punish them for their impertinence by taking the form of a most beautiful goddess. Fascinated by her beauty, the demons handed over the elixir to her, along with the right to decide who should receive it first. Vishnu in his disguise gave it to the gods, who immediately regained their strength and vitality. It was thus that the gods became immortal. The woman turned again into Vishnu—as even the gods cannot resist their own desire.

⌘⌘⌘⌘⌘

PRECONCEPTION STORIES

I often ask people to imagine a pre-earthly cosmic journey to prepare themselves for birth. These stories are about a life before earthly incarnation. A middle-aged musician clearly described his earthly mission. He wrote: "I died a long time ago. Epochs passed and I continued on until I reached the sun, where I designed my ancestry and birth. I climbed through and beyond, and experienced the joy of reunion with the cosmos." His saga ended: "Then I returned to Earth and found my way here, where you see me now."

Persian-Iranian teachers, Platonic philosophers, and Tibetan masters all report pre-earthly journeys, during which human spirits gather the necessary forces to fulfill earthly tasks. It is as if all humanity is brought before great looms and given the possibility of choosing the very colors and experiences needed to weave the tapestry of the life ahead. From a vastly creative overview, we descend into our bodies. Some colors are dark and disturbing, others more radiant. In descending, our vision narrows and we drink the waters of forgetfulness. When earthly colors wash over us, we forget from whence we came and how we have brought earthly conditions upon ourselves.

A depressed woman who was often ill struggled for years to understand why she had been born into a deeply troubled family and had to endure much sexual abuse. In one of my healing storytelling groups, she found her creative core of courage and decided to write a story about her soul's journey before birth.

> Once there was a human soul who lived on a faraway star as an angel. She considered going to live on Earth to be born to a particular couple. She looked down from her timeless perspective and saw that many who lived there had a strange soul-illness. Some were so malnourished in soul that they were like Chronos, an insatiable Greek god who ate his own children. The children of these parents, when they grew up, would often eat their own children's souls, too. And so the earth-parent sickness would pass from one generation to another. She observed multitudes of earth children suffering in great darkness. The human-angel longed to do something to help with this. As she looked down to Earth, she decided to join a family in their darkness and suffering, and try to help.

An angel in her story agreed to accompany her. This guardian angel said that she would sometimes forget and feel very alone, and sometimes she would remember that she was not alone. In her story, the human soul passed through all of the planetary realms to gather the strengths and qualities she would need to endure her mission on Earth. This story gave much relief to this deeply depressed woman. Tapping into her creativity awakened joy and self-affirmation as she expressed to the storytelling group what she felt was her deepest soul's intention: to learn how to relieve her own and all possible human suffering.

Holy and Carnal Love

Holy longings that apply with equal relevance to sexual relationships and meditation are: *Let there be no distraction. Let not the universe withhold itself from me.* Sexuality can bring us close to the mysteries of suffering and death, as well as fill us with the joys of union. It is not surprising that the seductive realms of desire, through which we all must pass again and again, inspire many stories, such as this one, about carnal love leading to greater enlightenment.

⁕⁓⁕⁓⁕

The Buddha and the Courtesan

Once in the time of the Buddha, there was a courtesan renowned for her beauty and amorous services. Her clients came to her from far and wide and she ran a most successful household with many servants. But one day, the Buddha himself came to speak near where she lived. She sat at the back of the crowd, her face exquisitely veiled. As she listened to the Buddha, his presence touched her more deeply than any man before had ever done, and from that moment on she decided that she would live her life differently. She put all of her wealth and her servants at the service of those in need, sent away her many clients, and devoted herself to helping the poor.

Nearby there lived a young man amongst the followers of the Buddha. This devotee came to her door one day with a begging bowl. In that moment, he fell hopelessly in love with her, returning to her house whenever he could to catch even a glimpse of her. She attended to him personally, bearing him food.

Not long afterward, she caught a curious illness. Despite the aid of doctors, she died. The Buddha, knowing of her former occupation, asked the king of that province for her body. This wish was granted, and the Buddha ordered that her body be displayed naked on a cremation pyre at the edge of the river for all to see. Of course, the news spread far and near and many came to witness this remarkable sight, amongst them the many men who had enjoyed her favors, and their wives who knew of her former reputation.

The Buddha would welcome them, offering her body for sale. "You who paid so much for her favors in the past, which one of you will take her now?"

In the heat, her body was rapidly decomposing. Flies and maggots swarmed upon her, and still the Buddha offered her for sale. Each day, he lowered the price, until he was prepared to give her away for free. The young lover came every day, weeping amongst the crowd. Soon he was the only one who remained. The Buddha beckoned for him to come close, and gazing at his face with loving compassion, reached out and wiped away his tears. It was only then that the young man understood the teachings of the Buddha about the impermanence of everything, even the beauty of women. With her life's work completed, the Buddha released her body to the fires.

༄༅།

Tyrants and Sirens

When sexuality is detached from higher morality and the heart's wisdom, it has merely its own compelling self-interest. Voluptuaries can be fickle and honeymoons do not always lead to enduring relationships. Hollywood siren Zsa Zsa Gabor, with her Hungarian accent, quick wit, and beguiling curves, attracted nine husbands and countless lovers. She herself quipped, "How many husbands have I had? Do you mean, apart from my own?" Elizabeth Taylor has had at least seven marriages, colored by dramatic concerns about paternity, jealousy, and polyandry.

Lust spins both comic and tragic story lines in all cultures. It provoked the Trojan War. Hester Prynn's luscious innocence in Hawthorne's *The Scarlet Letter* caused her lover's death. Homer's *Odyssey* portrays sirens that awaken oceanic desires that waste life away to barren death. The hero of this huge mythic saga, Odysseus, wanted to experience fully for himself the power of their attraction and singing. He prepared himself well before coming to the realm of these sirens. He asked his crew to bind him with strong ropes to the mast of their boat and no matter how much he howled for freedom, to keep him tied. They were required to seal up their ears. When the great hero cried out with the desperation of adolescent desire to respond to these sirens, his men kept his command, and so all were able to pass safely through that very dangerous part of the ocean of desire.

Surviving and Remembering Our Desires

Stories help us find perspective on even our most disturbing feelings. Everyone has tales to tell of overwhelming passions and desires. If and when we have survived, it can be a relief to give these episodes an airing once in a while. The sexual type loves more than occasional open discussion of sexual encounters. Before you know it, they will draw you with seductive persistence into sharing your own most intimate sexual experiences. At the request of a friend, I held a workshop on a cold Saint Valentine's Day for people to turn their most excruciating romantic adventures into stories. The laughter and tears and honesty were cleansing for us all. Maturity requires that we gain perspectives on very disconcerting passions—jealousy, pride, and other passions that rouse in sexual heat. To spur us on, one story told during the workshop was "The Green Bottle."

A man who was very jealous of his wife became suspicious of everything she did. If she brushed her hair in front of the mirror, he was sure it was for another man. If she wore a lovely dress, he was certain it was for someone else. He could not bear to let her out of his sight for even a moment. Finally, his feelings reached such a feverish pitch that she threatened to leave him unless he changed his ways. So he went to see a healer who prescribed a remarkable cure.

"Take this little green bottle," she said. "Whenever you are filled with feelings of jealousy, simply blow over its mouth, and your wife will disappear for a while. No harm will come to her, and you both will find rest from this torment. When you want her back, just blow twice."

Though doubtful, the man was prepared to try her remedy. Very soon he had his first opportunity. He blew, and voilà! she was gone. She found herself in a little green room, complete with everything she needed. When the husband summoned her with two blows on the bottle, she reappeared, somewhat confused, but with no memory of where she had been. The husband was delighted. At last he felt he had this monster under control.

Life improved to the extent that he sometimes felt confident to step out and leave her alone. So it happened one day that she discovered the green bottle as she was standing at the window overlooking the street. At that moment, a remarkably handsome man happened to be strolling by. "Phew," she exclaimed, breathing over the bottle. To her astonishment, the man disappeared. Not long after, the husband returned, as did his suspicions.

He quickly grabbed the bottle and blew over its mouth. Needless to say, his wife found lively companionship in the green room. When the husband had regained his composure, he blew twice and there before him his worst nightmare came true. Gentle reader, end this story as you are so inclined.

Transformational Storytelling
Genital Affirmation
I am love desiring love.

Basic Genital Story Dynamic
Moody frivolity becomes passionate devotion.

Genital Protagonists and Antagonists
Genital protagonists (characters who support genital health) are dignified like gods and goddesses, desirous, caressing, caring, uninhibited, gracious, and amiable.

Genital antagonists (characters who express genital dysfunction) are careless, self-damaging, empty-headed, conceited, fickle, frantic, seductive, and exploitative of others.

Basic Story Elements

Myths and stories often resonate with specific internal processes. This reliable pattern invokes well-being and resilience in every cell of your body:

Setting Out: The protagonist sets out in quest of greater love, strength, justice, wisdom, and happiness.

Trouble: One or more obstacles and/or antagonists interfere with the journey.

Help: Wise and benevolent help comes, often giving a gift.

Positive Ending: The protagonist fulfils the quest with joy and celebration.

SUMMONING YOUR STORYTELLER

Each performance for genital-strong storytellers is an act of public lovemaking. They invite their audience to enjoy the delights of amorous companionship and welcome them to experience both physical and emotional closeness. They want the audience to make themselves comfortable even before a word is said. They are seductive without apology. Their speech is breathy, enticing, unhurried. The stories they choose to tell tend to be neither "nice" nor overly intellectual as they heat up the emotional zone. They may feed a baby at their breast as they tell their stories, which may include balls, guts and ovaries. As they speak, a sense of excitement brings the audience toward blissful new awareness, similar to being in love.

Exercises to Explore and Balance the Realm of the Genitals

The power of holy desire. Referring to the qualities listed, set a clock for seven minutes and write a story in which a caring protagonist meets and transforms an antagonist.

In the myth of Isis and Osiris, the goddess Isis searches the world for the dismembered body of her beloved. She finds every part of Osiris, except his penis. This she forms out of cedarwood and gold, whispering over it words of power so that in the next world it will engender blessings. Take pieces of wood or clay and shape the sexual organs of each gender separately, then bring them into a sublime artistic relationship.

Mirror, mirror, on the wall. Stand before a full-length mirror. As you behold yourself, thank all that makes it possible for you to be as wonderful as you are. Out of modesty or natural revulsion, you may not like this exercise at first, but soon you will see others with new eyes, too. For inspiration, read William Carlos Williams's poem "Danse Russe" and Maya Angelou's poem "Phenomenal Woman."

The matchmaker. Imagine a village where a highly skilled matchmaker lives. She or he entices you (or someone) to reveal the full spectrum of your attractive traits, to see your body as a temple, an architectural wonder, every part a shrine. The matchmaker writes these traits on a beautiful scroll with golden edges and posts this scroll for all to see in the village square. The story goes on from there. It must have an ecstatic ending.

Homage to love. Plan an event in which the protagonists, you and your true love, will be the center of attention. Nothing of you need be hidden. All who gaze on you, even the plants and animals, are fortunate to be close to you; they feel both excited and satisfied in your presence. All of your guests place gifts at your feet. Each of your actions and words thrills your guests with pleasure and comfort.

Erotica. Healthy sexuality gives a strong sense of being the center of attraction, whether softly enveloping or asserting. Ransack your memories of your own personal sexual adventures. Perhaps concentrate on one that is hilariously embarrassing. Write it down with voluptuous resolve as a story, using third person "he" or "she," rather than "I." Then share your story with a trusted friend. As you read, enjoy the mating dance between your voice and your emotions.

Expanding Genital Awareness Through Dance, Music, and Yoga

Dance

Standing upright, allow your hips to move freely in figure eights. Dance from your hips as if you are responding with all your parts in a continuous stream to the intimate emotional needs of your most beloved.

Music

Strauss, Dance of the Seven Veils from *Salome*

Puccini, O mio babbino caro from *Gianni Schicchi*

Tchaikovsky, *Swan Lake* Overture

Saint Saens, *Romance Opus 37*

Wagner, *Tristan and Isolde*

Yoga asanas (Sanskrit names in italics)

Full Forward Bend *(Paschimothanasana)*

Sit-Up Reclining Bound Angle *(Supta Baddha Konasana)*

Hip flexor *(Supta Ardha Padmasana)*

Happy Baby *(Apanasana)*

16

Cultured Thinker: The Brain

Under the bony dome of every human skull, the whole universe in miniature learns to reflect upon itself. In subtle memory centers, every human brain knows the origin of the universe out of which it is formed and its evolutionary saga. A version of the human brain was there from the beginning, before time and space. Amassed and organized from cosmic and earthly influences, the brain creates reflections of itself and myths are born. In ancient Nordic myth, Odin squints from a godly height as he observes creation from his seat at the top of Yggdrasil, the Tree of Life. In Greek mythology, Athene springs in brilliant regalia from the head of Zeus to preside over the emerging intellect of Athens.

Enclosed as it is within the private and often foggy night of the cranium, the human brain seeks light. On its lone height above everyone's body, it allows us freedom to think our individual thoughts and to brighten up dull and murky ones. It has a sometimes mournful enthusiasm for reflecting on all things. In universities around the globe, minds concentrate together with natural gleaming curiosity, often seeking the universal truths that reside in particular realms of knowledge. Hungry convoluted gray matter learns to remember and to know that we know. The brain, seemingly for its own enjoyment, sets up halls of myriad minute dancing mirrors that can light up within as it accumulates its own archive of impressions and memories. Thoughts visit us like flocks of birds to a nesting ground or bees to a hive.

THE INTRICATE PLAYFUL BODY-BRAIN

The brain is made up of nerves and glands and is the coolest part of the body. Within a few weeks after they form in the embryo, brain cells are incapable of regeneration. Their mission is to hold thoughts and to move them around. Nerves extend from each organ to the brain, creating reflective brightness that can feel chilly in contrast with blood that continuously radiates warmth throughout the body. Yet as the nerves and brain together work toward mastering situations, facts, and data, the brain can work even at the speed of light—and ultimately experience a condition of enlightenment. In his book *It Was on Fire When I Lay Down on It,* Robert Fulghum recounts a story told to him by a wise man from the island of Crete. As a child this man had found a broken piece of a mirror. He could not find any other pieces, but he kept the one he did find. As he played with the fragment of the mirror, he was fascinated to see that he could reflect sunlight with it into dark places. It became a game he loved. Turning the mirror at an angle, he especially enjoyed shining light into the darkest places he could find, where the sun would otherwise never shine. As he grew up, the man realized that his childhood game was a metaphor for his life, and that he was a fragment of a mirror whose whole design and shape he did not know. He realized that truth, understanding, and knowledge could shine in dark places within and around him if he reflected them.

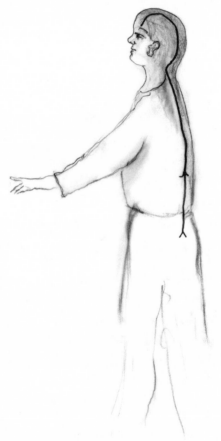

The Governing Vessel

Plato described the brain-mind as a prisoner in a cave who sees mere shadows of reality moving on the wall. As it reflects on everything from its lofty position at the top of the body, the light-reflecting, nerve-rich brain-mind tends to disconnect from the body. Although the grand human mind includes all the intelligence of the body, various parts of the brain within it can think they are the whole mind. It is not surprising that the heady brain-mind tends to think it is superior. Apollo's words resound today: "Know thyself." As it organizes and compartmentalizes thoughts, the brain-mind strives to know itself and bring about a more enlightened culture, yet it often fails to notice that every part of the body is informed with amazing intelligence, too. This intelligence lacks, however, the brain's special ability of conscious reflection that can "lift off" and create television and computer screens, and an endless array of other brainy, rather disembodied versions of reality.

Hence, in Chinese medicine, the brain is balanced with the ever-challenging, resplendent, and very much less conscious sexuality at the opposite pole of the torso. The upper brain pole connects with the pelvic cavity through the meridian known in Chinese medicine as the Governing Vessel. This energy line ascends from the tip of the tailbone along the spinal column that sends out thirty-one pairs of spinal cord nerves to communicate with every part of the body. Gathering energy from the whole body, it penetrates into the brain. A branch continues over the top of the head and across the forehead and nose to end inside the upper gums. One way to stimulate this energetic pattern is to stand upright. As you place one hand gently on your tailbone, lift your chin slightly with the fingers of your other hand, and carefully walk about, thoughtfully observing the world.

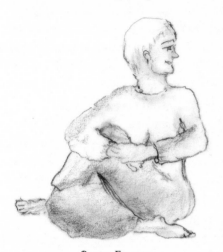

Brain Exercise

Another simple physical exercise to stimulate a flow of brain energy is to place your right hand on your left knee or left shoulder. Straighten your spine and lift your head slightly, turning it gently to the right as your torso resists from the left. In the annals of human evolution, curiosity strengthens noses and heightens brows. As you breathe and relax, your nose will tend to tilt upward and your brainstem may slowly bloom into your brow with a new electrical charge. Then change hands and turn your head slightly upward and to the left. This simple spinal twist lifts cerebral spinal fluid, and activates cranial polarities. It sets in motion an endless stream of paradoxical thoughts. It will stretch and activate your larynx, and you may feel an impulse from this cerebral energy to vocalize your most perplexing questions.

Try standing side by side with a partner or, better yet, in a circle with several others. Place right hands over left, each person tugging gently on the hands at either side. Breathe deeply as you straighten your spine and contract the back of your legs. Gently turn your head over each shoulder, and hold each position for a while, tilting your nose slightly upward. This exercise produces a distinctive feeling of superiority, autonomy, and enlightened serenity. When your head has returned to front and center, then let your hands drop to your sides, and notice how your attention has changed. The whole group together may feel a quite enjoyable "upper deck" heady view of the world.

A CURIOUS NUT

The human brain resembles the beautifully connected two-lobed kernel of a walnut. When we are born, this wondrous nut within us has already formed and ripened on the venerable Tree of Knowledge for countless ages. With infinite potential, it dove as embryo into your mother's center of gravity to begin its quest for freedom of thought. Neatly crammed, orderly, and eager to shine forth and add to its already vast contents, it glistens for a lifetime within the hard protective shell of the skull. Once I saw a wry storyteller introduce an evening of his brilliantly researched tales about trees by knocking affectionately on his forehead. "Here, have a taste of my nut," he said.

With great good taste, healthy brain personalities delight in sharing what they have mastered in the thought world. Many a vigorously buoyant teacher, lawyer, physician, or politician inhabits this realm. Head-dominant folk enjoy the stir of brainstorms and other brilliant activities. For relaxation, they may turn to the tickle and challenge of "brain teasers" and puzzles, or to mastering musical instruments. With spectacled, sometimes dreamy faces and infinite good will, in a cloud of unknowing, they may brood on questions, linking old thoughts with fresh ones, making fascinating connections. As they attempt to keep up with all the experts in their field and to contribute to the latest unfolding knowledge, their clarifications often serve to stimulate others.

Those who live primarily in their heads are attracted to environments where intriguing research is going on. They enjoy brooding in ivory towers and gathering in elite groves of academe, experimental laboratories, and research institutes set apart from the more chaotic hurly-burly of life. Such ivory towers allow them uninterrupted time to observe, and to think thoughts through to clarity. Walter Russell, a twentieth-century Renaissance man, wrote, "I learned to cross the threshold of my studio with reverence, as though I am entering a shrine to the Universal Thinker."

Many a brilliantly urbane psychiatrist, novelist, short story writer, or essayist roams in a study abounding in open books, grazing and gleaning from them with great enjoyment. Imperial learners, they acquire volumes of information, and create libraries, bookstores, or laboratories to surround themselves serenely and powerfully with questions, inventions, and the written word. Other brain-focused folk bemuse themselves with concealed esoteric, symbolic levels of meaning, which they feel moved to master. Intellectuals sometimes revel in literary criticism and whodunit thrillers that blend the antagonistic themes of the skin with intense mental acuity. The brain also becomes an enclave where spies and other "undercover" secret agents learn their trade and pursue furtive investigations. Cheerfully polite private detectives, such as Conan Doyle's Sherlock Holmes and Agatha Christie's Miss Marple, solve mind-boggling mysteries, making connections where others have not, moving about skillfully. As cartographers, they measure the world; as reporters, they wield their third-eye cameras.

When brainy folk relax to think things out, they often play with data, which for them is pleasurable. They laugh at being called "genius" when others are baffled by their skills and methods. As they map out work to be done and deftly proceed, they often impress others by seeing what others do not, as in the following story.

There was once a teacher who always had an apt story for every occasion. One of his students asked him, "Master, how is it you always have the right tale?"

The master replied, "Well, let me tell you a story. There was once a man who wished to become the greatest marksman in the world. He applied himself until there seemed to be no one in the world who could better him. But one day he was walking though the countryside and he passed a barn on the sides of which were many targets, and in the center of each target, an arrow. He immediately inquired of the farmer, 'What splendid marksman is responsible for this?' The farmer introduced him to his son. 'Tell me,' said the visitor, 'I am a celebrated marksman, yet never have I seen such skill as this. How do you manage to hit the center each time?' 'It is easy,' the young man replied. 'I shoot my arrow at the barn, and then I paint a circle around it.'"

Many a mythic and fairy-tale hero exercises similar efficiency, like the nimble hero of "The Valiant Little Tailor" who outwits angry giants with ease. His cousin, "The Cunning Little Tailor," also found in the Grimms' collection, easily guesses all the riddles of a proud and headstrong princess and, "happy as a wood lark," marries her.

Cautionary Tales for Scatterbrains

To attain pleasant endings, stories of many lands caution us against mere harebrained plans. A head that is totally wrapped up in itself may fail to see clearly practical matters beyond its own ideas. An old English tale shows how thoughts can drift dreamily away from practical action.

Johnny and the Hare

Johnny was out walking one fine day when he spied a hare sitting under a bush. He thought, "What luck! Here's me and I'll catch this hare, and then I'll sell him. With that money I can get a young sow, I reckon; and I'll feed her up on scraps, and she'll bring me twelve piglets. The piglets when they've grown, they'll have twelve piglets each. And when they've grown, they'll bring me a barnload of pork. I'll sell the pork, and I'll buy a little house for my mother to live in. Then I can get married myself. I'll marry the farmer's daughter. We'll have two sons; and I'll work them hard and pay them little. They'll oversleep in the morning, and I'll have to give them a shout to raise them. 'Get up you lazy beggars!' I'll say. 'The cows need milking.'" Johnny fell so in love with his big ideas that he really did shout, "Get up, you lazy beggar!" And the hare that had been sitting under the bush took fright at the row Johnny was making and ran off across the fields and Johnny never did catch it; and his money, pigs, house, wife, farm, and children were lost, all because of that.

A BRAIN SUBLIMELY FOCUSED CREATES MIRACLES

Although intellect can leave us detached and cold, it can also help us master challenging circumstances. Concentrated cerebral pleasures and mental effort can also result in astonishing leaps of self-development. Many of the greatest fairy tales portray the attainment of true human dignity against great odds. One of the wisest of the old stories collected by the Grimm brothers is called "The Donkey." The story was already popular in late medieval times and a stone carving illustrating it was placed at the south cornice of Chartres Cathedral when it was originally built. To this day, you can see there the same stone image of a merry donkey playing a lute, an emblem of the soul's determination to evolve and to create harmony.

The Donkey

Once upon a time there lived a king and a queen who were rich and had everything they wanted, but no children. The queen lamented over this day and night, and said, "I am like a field on which nothing grows." At last God fulfilled her wish. But when the child came into the world, it did not look like a human child, but instead was a little donkey. When the mother saw him, her lamentations and outcries began in earnest; she said that she would far rather have no child at all than have a donkey.

But the king protested, "No, since God has sent him, he shall be my son and heir, and after my death he shall sit on the royal throne, and wear the kingly crown."

The donkey therefore was brought up as a prince, and as he grew, his ears grew high and straight and he was of a merry disposition. He jumped about, played, and took special pleasure in music. One day he went to a celebrated musician and said, "Teach me your art, so that I may play as well as you do."

The little royal donkey completely ignored the limitations of his body as he pursued his beloved music. By the end of the story, accomplished musicianship had permeated his rough animal body and he had thoroughly transformed himself into the handsome human prince that he truly was. In perfect happiness, he became the worthy husband to a king's daughter and, in the end, a king in his own right.

A PATH TO ENLIGHTENED BRAIN DEVELOPMENT

The brain has the capacity to connect with every part of us and be a conscious receptor for each organ. Yet whoever becomes absorbed in vortices of bright brain activity often discovers an ability to ignore emotion. Brain-dominant folks may work on something quite privately, and for indefinite periods of time tune out the feelings and social interactions of others. Their body may seem to be a vaguely interesting appendage to clothe nicely and tend with respect, but nevertheless a rather strange reality that moves around underneath the dominant lights above. As they work their primary territory, such people can have quite a puzzled relation with what is going on down under. The long ancient journey down to the body can be avoided as they entertain thoughts and pursue the balm of reason. Approaching problems from above, they may sometimes seem haughty to others. Curiously pleased with themselves, less emotionally involved with visceral life, they tend to smell even battle from aloft and to take it on primarily as a mental curiosity. A friend of mine always referred to his debonair and brainy father as "the governor." This elderly gentleman, as he was reflecting coolly on his impressive biography, said, "Curiosity was the major drawing force in every area of my life, including sex."

Intellectuals often see an overview and often take a mournful attitude toward what they observe of human behavior. When they feel compassion in their hearts, they may devotedly serve others. They can shine like a lighthouse for those whose thoughts are floundering at sea. With clear thinking, they can give noble hope to all, whether the homeless, the addicted, the confused corporate executive, or the blue-collar worker. Whether they are alone or with a select few, when they step forth from library, desk, or armchair, they can be fonts of knowledge and enlightenment for others. Though some may drain us with their talk, at their best they continue thinking with refined wit, providing an articulate tonic of poise and sophistication in an otherwise chaotic world of impulse and desire. They revel in the self-fertilizing fluidity of living ideas.

In every country of the world, "brains" are busy enlightening others. Some create ferociously brilliant satires and caricatures, as did H. H. Munro, better known as Saki, with his acerbic tales of upper-crust English society. Some, like Goethe's Faust, seek to master all knowledge, yet dream of being distracted by luxury, wealth, and the satisfaction of sexuality. Some appear to be a special sort of absentminded space and time traveler. The star mind glimpses and sometimes realizes its own magnificence. A very evolved few with a greatly expanded capacity for reflecting reality offer a cosmic story. Sri Aurobindo, Paramahansa Yogananda, and Rudolf Steiner were such persons. Immensely enlightened thinkers, they found within themselves the ability to shed light on every territory to which they turned.

TRUTH AND UNTRUTH

Brainy folk often have good-humored perspectives on their own lofty urges. As they try to free themselves from the body, they may be drawn more strictly into its laws. The stress of repressed emotion can drain bodily energies, causing twitching tics and other nervous disorders. Yet they can often chuckle at their difficulties relating to the more physical dimensions of reality, and make up witty stories. Anthony de Mello, a highly enlightened Jesuit priest, maintained his sanity, honesty, and good humor through collecting and sharing stories, such as this sardonic quest tale.

What Is Truth?

A man abandoned all his worldly life to go in search of truth. He searched up the hills and down the valleys. He went into small villages and large towns, into forests and along the coasts of the wide sea, into grim wastes and lush meadows. One day atop a high mountain in a small cave, he thought he had at last found one who knew all that he sought.

She was a wizened old woman with but a single tooth left in her head, and hair that hung down onto her shoulders in greasy strands. Her skin was wizened and leathery, but her voice was lyrical and pure. The wanderer decided that he had reached his destination. He stayed a long time with her and learned all that she had to teach. At last he stood at the mouth of the cave, ready to depart for home.

He said, "Lady Truth," for so he called her, "You have taught me so much. Is there anything I can do for you?" She put her head to one side and considered. Then she raised a withered finger. "When you speak of me," she said, "tell them I am young and beautiful."

LOST AND FOUND IN THE LABYRINTH

When thinkers are physically sensitive and vulnerable in body and soul, knowledge is their power. Their towering thoughts provide a crust of protection. They are willing to give up everything else to attain command of their subject. They seek to master reality by drawing all their energy up into their brains to manipulate their sense impressions and maneuver through their days and nights with their abstract, symbolic thinking. A thin-skinned, sensitive man attended one of my healing story workshops.

He spent long hours every day depressed and hunched at computers, brilliantly translating scientific texts into several languages. When he was reminded that the higher mind includes the whole body, he complained abstractly, "Overpowering forces rob the human core before it has had a chance to blossom. I know a human being should be able to respond with feelings to children, to other people's suffering and joys, and to one's own life."

The story he made up during the workshop surprised and fascinated him. It drew him down into the great power of his body. Soon after he wrote and shared the following story, he reported with joy that he had started a successful relationship with a very loving woman.

Long ago, in the Kingdom of the North, there lived a king and a queen. At last a son was born to them, and their joy was great. The people set their hopes upon him, for special signs were on him: a high brow, deep-blue-black eyes, and a walrus-shaped birthmark on his abdomen. Years passed and the lad grew radiant and wise. At night, he spoke with the stars that shone down through the roof of his ice palace. Finally, he reached the age when young men go out to seek their spirit-calling. Those who returned from these quests alive became men and leaders.

The prince saw his father's counselors pointing to his downy cheeks and weak muscles and heard them muttering, "The boy is too soft to face the dangers of the quest. What if he should fall under the spell of the walrus king? Indeed he might lose his heart, or his life."

The prince stood at the window of the ice palace watching as the other young men prepared for their journeys. Their strapping shoulders and taut arms shone in the sun as they bound their belongings to their sleds and departed. One by one, they walked out alone across the icy expanse. In the dim light before dawn, the prince slipped out of the palace and hastened to the edge of the sea. Stepping into a small boat, he took the oars. The next morning, the anguished news spread throughout the kingdom. The young prince was gone.

For three days and three nights, he paddled, but he did not find the other men. On the morning of the fourth day, he heard a call in the distance. Thinking the hunting party was there, he pointed his boat toward a great mountain of ice. He stepped out and began to climb. At the top of the mountain was a yawning blue crevasse, and out of it came a great trumpeting. He took a step to peer farther, but the midday sun had melted the ice.

He slipped and down and down he slid, how long and how far, he could not say. When his feet finally touched solid ground, he was surrounded by grunting walruses. Rough warm bellies pushed and jostled him through a dark tunnel in the ice. At length they came out into a high domed room where, on a couch of blue ice, the walrus king reclined.

Suddenly, the young prince felt the heavy blow of a walrus tail between his shoulder blades, and in a strange flickering light, he fell. When he awoke, his heart was not his own. It was the heart of a walrus. Along with the yelping walruses, he clambered out of the cave onto the ice. The next moment harpoons flew through the air and the walruses around him fell grunting and shrieking. A hunter came closer. The prince recognized the hunter and tried to speak to him, but all that came out of his throat were walrus grunts.

The hunter cast a heavy net of wet rope over him and called to his comrades, "This one has offered himself for the sacrifice. Look at the beauty in his eyes! Do not kill him."

When the hunting party returned with the walrus as captive, the kingdom was in mourning, for they believed the prince was lost. The hunters tied their walrus catch to a stout post in an ice pen. The curious pointed, admiring his sleek body and blue-black eyes. He called and looked at them imploringly. His squeals filled the skies.

In the evening, a princess of that realm walked by to see the walrus of which everyone was speaking. As she approached, the blue-black eyes and the imploring squeal touched her heart. She opened the door to the pen. Leaning closer, her eyes were drawn to a deep blue mark on his abdomen that had the shape of a walrus: the royal insignia. Warm tears burst from her eyes. Three nights long, the princess wept over the enchanted prince. Three nights long, her hot salty tears streamed over his head and down his tough hide. After the first night, his skin began to soften. After the second night, his thick walrus blubber began to melt. At the end of the third night, her tears touched his walrus heart and it became a human heart again. In the morning, the prince stepped forth. There was great rejoicing at his transformation and the wedding that soon took place.

Holding on to the Golden Thread

As the brain attempts to detach from the larger self, it moves us slightly out of our physical bodies. This can produce a vast array of images that have been generated by repressed feelings. Desire, fear, and terror can rear their ominous heads in stories, as in life, until a higher power offers loving connection to better worlds. Then the brain is able to reintegrate with the body and soul, as in this ancient Greek myth:

❦❦❦❦

The Labyrinth

Minos, ancient king of Crete, mourned for his son, who had been sent on a quest by the king of Athens and killed by a bull. He asked the great architect and inventor Daedalus to construct a labyrinth or maze of underground tunnels and chambers. In retribution for the death of his son, Minos asked that fourteen young Athenian men and women once every year be sent as food for a monstrous Minotaur that was captive in the subterranean brain. When the great Athenian hero Theseus entered the darkness of the labyrinth, Ariadne, King Minos's daughter, out of her passionate concern for his safety, gave him a ball of thread. He fastened the thread to the door as he entered the maze. It unwound as he went. He descended boldly, certain that he could find his way out again. In the depths of the dark, he came upon the unsuspecting Minotaur asleep. At last Theseus was able to crush the life out the monster. The dead head swayed slowly as Theseus lifted himself up from the terrific struggle and found the thread again, just where he had dropped it. With the thread, the way back was clear. Ariadne was waiting for him and joined him on the ship filled with rejoicing Athenians.

❦❦❦❦

A version of this subterranean labyrinth shines brightly on the floor of Chartres Cathedral and at numerous sacred sites around the world. Countless pilgrims walk these labyrinths slowly to find balance, quell their darkest fears, and comfort their souls with prayer.

FACING THE MONSTER HEAD

The destructive potential of the brain is portrayed in another vivid Greek myth of the Gorgon Medusa.

A jealous king wanted more than anything in the world to have the head of this goddess with snaky locks and the deadly power to terrorize all living beings and turn them to stone when they looked at her. A hero named Perseus longed to conquer this force, too, and the goddess Pallas Athena helped him. Athena gave him the shield of polished bronze that covered her heart, saying, "Look into this when you attack the Gorgon. You will be able to see her in it, as in a mirror, and so avoid her deadly power."

With this new power of magic, Perseus accomplished the impossible. He kept his head and protected his heart in the presence of a horrifying destructive power. With the reflective observation of a scientist, his eyes fixed fully on the shield, he seized and severed the monster's head. Then he dropped it into his silver wallet, and with Hermes ever at his side to protect him, went flying onward, swift as thought.

THE LUCIFERIC BRAIN

From one point of view, the Internet is a small experimental manipulation of the magnitude of reflective power in the human brain. The ancient Indian myth of Indra's net speaks of a vast net of mirrors strung across the entire cosmos, each mirror reflecting all the others. Yet transcendent reflection can become blocked, and fearsome shadows gain appalling strength. In the Apocryphal Christian tradition, the angel Lucifer portrays the mind in its self-reflective pride, fascinated by its own light, denying any source of light other than his own. The story of Lucifer's pride is replayed again and again. Sometimes, as we turn to our private egocentric thoughts, an enchanting power removes us from the light's ultimate Source. The wisdom imbuing the whole of Creation tends to shrink and descend within us to a private self-centered agenda.

❧❦❧❦❧

Lucifer's Fall

God gazed upon the brightness of Creation. All the heavens rang with celestial music. Angels descended tirelessly to earth and rose heavenward again. But finally one of the greatest angels sent tremors throughout the heavenly realms. This light-bearing angel made his way through Heaven, saying to lesser angels, "Help me build a throne and I will sit upon it and be your God. My throne will be the highest throne of all. To my throne you may always come." A gray cloud hovered before his forehead and his heart. Many hosts of angels were frightened at these words. Others liked Lucifer's enticing power so much that they agreed.

The archangel Michael observed what Lucifer was doing and warned the Supreme.

At last the Supreme spoke: "I will give him a new shining heart. If he will not receive this heart, he shall have his throne, but not in Heaven. If he refuses to heed my words, cast him out of Heaven."

But Lucifer went on stirring angels. These angels ceased their singing and instead their voices shouted in confusion.

At last, lightning flashed from Michael's sword as he struck against the wall of Heaven, and through the gash made by the sword, Lucifer and his angels fell. The colors of their garments and wings paled. They howled and wailed as they plunged into the depths of an unknown darkness. In this place of cold exile, they resigned themselves to making small fires out of their own light and forging, in the midst of their fires, a dark throne for Lucifer.

Where Michael closed the cleft in Heaven, a scar remained.

⁂

The Cramp of Paranoia

Lucifer set the stage for human development. Thinking of ourselves as separate from the rest of Creation, we focus on our own concerns. Pride and arrogance weaken the delicate web of thought that serves the whole body and soul. Daedalus constructed wings and covered them with wax and feathers to fly above the labyrinth of lower thoughts and desires. "I must try the wings," shouted his young son, Icarus, who set out impulsively, as we all do, insisting on his own ideas. The wax that held his winged apparatus aloft melted and he, too, fell into the darker depths of the human drama.

In stories and life, the sense-bound brain expands with possibilities, and eventually narrows to relieve the stress of expansion. A field of thought can turn weirdly against the thinker, who cries for companions, yet is too afraid to reach out to others. Fixed thoughts slip into destructive shadow realms. From a distance, strange glittering eyes peer back. Unable to access emotional needs, even kindness and caring may be suspect. Yet, eventually, with the help of the wisdom within and around us, we can learn to manage our thoughts and passions. Then the brilliantly narrow brainy ego gives way to more balanced use of gifts and abilities, and the story continues. Self-consciousness expands with humble joy, and sends us onward to grander realization.

TRANSFORMATIONAL STORYTELLING

Brain Affirmation

I am a reflection of all truth.

Basic Brain Story Dynamic

Undisciplined thinking transforms into elegant intelligence.

Brain Protagonists and Antagonists

Brain protagonists (characters who support brain health) are masterful, happy, adept, and rational. They are worldly, suave, eloquent, cheerful, honest, and self-governing in accordance with their high standards.

Brain antagonists (characters who express brain dysfunction) expect betrayal. They are jealous, devious, and nervous. Excessively independent, hostile, and argumentative, they tend toward lascivious secretiveness and paranoia.

Basic Story Elements

Myths and stories often resonate with specific internal processes. This reliable pattern invokes well-being and resilience in every cell of your body:

Setting Out: The protagonist sets out in quest of greater love, strength, justice, wisdom, and happiness.

Trouble: One or more obstacles and/or antagonists interfere with the journey.

Help: Wise and benevolent help comes, often giving a gift.

Positive Ending: The protagonist fulfils the quest with joy and celebration.

SUMMONING YOUR STORYTELLER

The storyteller who speaks predominantly from the intellect feels entitled to explore fields of knowledge serenely, and to bring encyclopedic mastery to the audience. Listeners are part of the storyteller's thought world. These storytellers warm to their subjects and enjoy the refinements and subtleties of their cogitations. Their clothing is appropriately cultured and understated, in keeping with their focus on thinking appropriately for the occasion. Their body feels distant and even incidental to whatever thought world they may inhabit. Their head remains quite still as they speak. Their gaze and attention are turned to the waves of thought unfolding from within them. Their voices ride on these waves of thought and memory, paying little heed to feelings. Such storytellers tend to expect an entirely cerebral response from their audiences.

Exercises to Explore and Balance the Realm of the Brain

Tale of the brain. Imagine a mastermind who is at work in a study or a laboratory. This person trusts that the universe is boundlessly intelligent. In a brief story, let this protagonist prevail over a very persistent antagonist.

Learning more. What learning would you like to acquire right now? What would be your perfect learning environment for mastering and playing with this new knowledge?

Encouraging right- and left-brain activity. Sometimes our heads say one thing and our hearts, or other parts, say another. Does your head sometimes feel like a small dimly lit lamp in a vast mansion? Tell of a time when your brain reasoning was entirely inadequate to what your larger self was telling you. Conversely, tell about a time when sudden clarity of thought saved you from the power of your feelings.

How did I know? The wisdom mind is malleable, mobile, and all-inclusive. It encompasses the whole body. Vast knowing is available to the brain when it is in the service of this vast wisdom mind. From time to time, an intriguing light turns on unexpectedly and we suddenly know and do things we had no idea we were capable of. This new capacity can dim again as quickly as it arrived. Describe an experience of this kind that you have had or witnessed in another's life.

Secret riddles and symbolic meanings. The brain enjoys analyzing and assigning coded messages to what it observes. Look at what is around you. Assign a symbolic meaning to what you see.

Make up a story to embellish a well-known riddle.

In a group, send one of you out of the room. The rest of you agree that when that person returns, he or she must give a little talk, and every time the person uses a certain word, such as "and," the whole group will look down. It is the task of the one speaking about the chosen subject to figure out the group's secret agreement.

Seeking to balance desire and detachment. Get as comfortable as possible, and recall with uninhibited abandon a highpoint in your romantic life. Then recover your poise, clasp your hands behind your back, and offer cool, brilliantly factual comments about this episode in your life.

Explore how the brain balances itself. Put on some vibrant music and dance with a real or imaginary partner. Move between intellectual poise and the sensual and voluptuous grace of your entire body.

Expanding Brain Awareness Through Dance, Music, and Yoga

Dance

Keep your torso still and move your head carefully in every direction. Bend forward slightly from above and, keeping your head still, explore space thoughtfully, first with your hands, then with your feet.

Music

Bach, *Goldberg Variations*
Clementi, *Etudes*
Shostakovich, Piano Trio no. 2 in E Minor

Yoga asanas (Sanskrit names in italics)

Seated Spinal Twist *(Arddha-Matsyendrasana)*
Shoulder Stand *(Sarvangasana)*
Fish Pose *(Matsyasana)*
Headstand *(Sirsasana)*

Afterword

Life invites us all to a perpetual healing festival. We heal as we access our own boundless potential. "Healing" means "wholeness." Around the world, we humans are on a grand adventure, endeavoring to live more harmoniously with one another and with ourselves. Similar as we all are in our bodily organization, I believe that in coming years the body will be recognized everywhere as the spiritual paradigm it is—a working model for a more enlightened and harmonious global human community. Our constant companion and inner teacher, our body, wherever we live on Earth, is always warmly announcing the theme of cooperation and conflict resolution.

How can we all learn to live respectfully with each other and ourselves, not only in theory and as an aspiration, but in fact? The spirited storyteller within you is a natural healer who loves to collaborate with the vast wisdom in every part of you. It enjoys helping you to hold the paradox of positive and negative impulses together in the same story in order to move you in the direction of greater well-being and global consciousness.

DEVELOPING MORE SPIRIT FOR EVOLUTION

Your whole body, with its vast supply of desire and memory, exuberance, and hope, is ready to support your transforming and evolving consciousness. As human beings, we are all designed to discover more of who we are. Every story in some way includes you and affects your total health. Some stories pull you toward your noblest humanity and others pull you down. Your body has been listening to you all your life and accumulating its own unique storehouse. Whether you intentionally make up a story or it makes up you, whatever is going on in your mind and emotional life at this moment is a story that you are telling your body. Each organ listens.

On our way toward greater awareness, our bodies enjoy certain stories and try to shut out others. Experiences fallen out of conscious memory and harbored in the body can eventually manifest as illness. Yet such blockages in healthy flowing energy can drive us into a more open and creative state. A slight or major breakdown of soul or body can resolve into new and expanded vitality. When organs go through pain and turbulence, when they block and dysfunction, we can easily forget that they are continuously nourished by their ultimate creative source, and by multitudes of energies from our surroundings that are playing through us.

In many ways, stories resemble the sheltering, vital flow and texture of our organs. Try telling your specific parts and your whole body a new story today. Stories can act as waking dreams, taking us into our wisdom mind and greater wholeness. As the life forces oscillating in a healing story shake and move us, healthy vitality is freed. Well-tuned stories can awaken more joy and well-being than we might ever have imagined. They can help us take hold of baffling episodes in our individual and collective lives that have been affecting our total health and that may have waited for years to be liberated.

Basic Story Dynamics

Heart   Anger becomes unconditional love.

Small Intestine   Self-denigration transforms into passion for truth, beauty, and goodness.

Liver   Emotionality matures into selfless service.

Gallbladder   Uncertainty transforms into devoted decisive action.

Large Intestine   Resistance turns into radiant accomplishments.

Lungs   Egocentric ambition becomes enlightened leadership.

Stomach   Addiction turns into brilliant nourishment of self and others.

Spleen & Pancreas   Codependency becomes conscious empathy.

Bladder   Self-display supports profound success for all.

Kidneys   Emptiness turns into joyous awareness.

Skin   Competition becomes companionable athletic vigor.

Pericardium   Condemnation becomes informed compassion.

Thymus   Destructiveness transforms into caring abundant generosity.

Appendix   Aloneness turns into prophetic wisdom.

Genitals   Moody frivolity becomes passionate devotion.

Brain   Undisciplined thinking transforms into elegant intelligence.

Affirming Your Body's Universal Story

Our bodies are built up from deep reserves of human endurance and vitality. Their communal wisdom is way ahead of our conscious minds. The diplomacy between our various parts tells us that, as sure as we breathe, we are all connected to one another and to the grand wholeness that sustains us. A wise elderly friend of mine always signed his letters A. V. P. He saw himself and everyone else as "Another Version of a Person." We are on the greatest of adventures, learning together to be human. When we accept our bodies as teachers, they bring us warmly and closely in touch with our potential for conscious personal and communal evolution. We are all part of one swiftly developing adventure story.

Affirmations instill spiritual ideals or goals in pithy, constructive statements. Affirmations are no less potent than stories. They activate universal attributes within and expand our consciousness. Each adds capacities to our total well-being. If you speak these affirmations silently or aloud, their meaning will evolve. You are invited to repeat these affirmations, focusing on one at a time, and in sequence as a whole.

Affirmations

Heart   My heart is filled with a ceaseless song of love.

Small Intestine   Beauty, truth, and love flame through me.

Liver   As I will to serve others, I am restored to life.

Gallbladder   I transform what interferes with life.

Large Intestine   Life perfects itself through me.

Lungs   I breathe the power of peace.

Stomach   I create catalytic movement for the benefit of all.

Spleen & Pancreas   I find within me the purity and sweetness I seek.

Bladder   I am a clear mirror.

Kidneys   All life connects within me.

Skin   Humanity shares one sacred skin.

Pericardium   I live compassionately, without blame.

Thymus   My life is a bounteous celebration.

Appendix   I transform to become enlightened.

Genitals   I am love desiring love.

Brain   I am a reflection of all truth.

The storyteller within you can draw together your whole being. As the body patiently provides the exquisitely organized foundation for your visions and words, may you awaken new integrity in your personal and communal story. You—like every one of us—hold the potential to discover all humanity alive within you. May we all see ourselves more fully in one another, and discover daily how to share a more conscious and caring adventure story

Suggested Reading

Aivanhov, Omraam Mikael, *Hope for the World*. France: Editions Prosveta, Frejus Cedex, 1987.

Aurobindo, Sri. *A Greater Psychology*. New York: Jeremy Tarcher, 2001.

_____. *Letters on Yoga 111*. Twin Lakes WI: Lotus Press, 1988.

Bark, Coleman. *The Essential Rumi*. Edison NJ: Castle Books, 1995.

Beinfield, Harriet, and Efrem Korngold. *Between Heaven and Earth: A Guide to Chinese Medicine*. New York: Ballantine, 1991.

Brody, Ed, Jay Goldspinner, Katie Green, and Rona Leventhal (eds). *Spinning Tales, Weaving Hope: Stories of Peace, Justice and the Environment*. Philadelphia: New Society, 1992.

Church, Dawson, Geralyn Gendreau, and Randy Peyser (eds). *Healing the Heart of the World*. Santa Rosa, CA: Elite Books, 2005.

Cook, Elizabeth. *The Ordinary and the Fabulous: An Introduction to Myths, Legends and Fairy Tales*. London: Cambridge University Press, 1969.

Cooley, Bob. *The Genius of Flexibility*. New York. Simon & Schuster, 2005.

Cox, Allison M., and David H. Albert (eds). *The Healing Heart: Families*. Gabriola Island, BC: New Society, 2003.

_____. *The Healing Heart: Communities*. Gabriola Island, BC: New Society, 2003.

Eden, Donna, with David Feinstein. *Energy Medicine*. New York: Jeremy Tarcher, 1998.

Emoto, Masaru. *The Secret Life of Water*. New York: Atria Books, 2005.

Feinstein, David, Donna Eden, and Gary Craig. *The Promise of Energy Psychology*. New York: Jeremy Tarcher, 2005.

Gendlin, Eugene. *Focus-Oriented Psychotherapy: A Manual for the Experiential Method*. New York: Guilford Press, 1996.

Grossinger, Richard. *Embryogenesis*. Berkeley, CA: North Atlantic Books, 1986.

Heriza, Nirmala. *Dr. Yoga*. New York: Jeremy Tarcher, 2004.

Husemann, Armin. *The Harmony of the Human Body: Musical Principles in Human Physiology*. Edinburg: Floris. 1994.

Iyengar, B. K. S. *Light on Yoga*. New York: Schocken Books, 1979.

Jocelyn, Beredene. *Citizens of the Cosmos*. New York: Continuum, 1981.

Johnson, Don Hanlon. *Body: Recovering Our Sensual Wisdom*. Berkeley, CA: North Atlantic Books, 1993.

Kane, Sean. *Wisdom of the Mythtellers*. Orchard Park, NY: Broadview Press, 1998.

Kaptchuk, Ted. *The Web That Has No Weaver*. Chicago: Contemporary Books, 2000.

Klocek, Dennis. *Seeking Spirit Vision*. Fair Oaks, CA: Rudolf Steiner College Press, 1998.

Ladinsky, Daniel. *I Heard God Laughing: Renderings of Hafiz*. Oakland CA: Mobius Press, 1996.

Lehrer, Warren. *Brother Blue*. Seattle, WA: Bay Press, 1995.

Lipton, Bruce. *The Biology of Belief*. Santa Rosa, CA: Elite Books, 2005.

Luby, Sue. *Hatha Yoga for Total Health*. Englewood Cliffs, NJ: Prentice-Hall, 1977.

Martin, Rafe. *The Hungry Tigress: Buddhist Legends and Jakata Tales*. Berkeley, CA: Parallax Press, 1990.

Murphy, Michael. *The Future of the Body*. Los Angeles: JP Tarcher, 1992.

Pearce, Joseph Chilton. *The Biology of Transcendence*. Rochester, VT: Park Street Press, 2002.

Pearsall, Paul. *The Heart's Code: Tapping the Wisdom and Power of Our Heart Energy*. New York: Broadway, 1998.

Pert, Candace. *Molecules of Emotion: The Science Behind Mind-Body Medicine*. New York: Simon and Schuster, 1997.

Richards, M.C. *Toward Wholeness: Rudolf Steiner Education in America*. Middletown CT: Wesleyan University Press, 1980.

Riso, Don, and Russ Hudson. *Personality Types: Using the Enneagram for Self-Discovery*. Boston: Houghton Mifflin, 1996.

Sahasranama, Sri Lalita. *The Thousand Names of the Divine Mother*. San Ramon, CA: Mata Amritanandamayi Center, 1996.

Steiner, Rudolf. *Curative Education: Twelve Lectures for Doctors and Curative Teachers*. London: Rudolf Steiner Press, 1972.

_____. *Eurythmy as Visible Speech*. London: Rudolf Steiner Press, 1983.

_____. *Introducing Anthroposophical Medicine*. Great Barrington, MA: Steiner Books, 2007.

_____. *Study of Man*. New York: Anthroposophic Press, 1947.

Takahashi, Takeo. *Atlas of the Human Body*. New York: HarperPerennial, 1994.

Thie, John F., and Matthew Thie. *Touch for Health*. Camarillo, CA: DeVorss, 2005.

Ulanov, Ann & Barry. *Transforming Sexuality: The Archetypal World of Anima and Animus*. Boston MA: Shambhala, 1994.

Wigmore, Ann. *Why Suffer? How I Overcame Illness and Pain Naturally*. Wayne, NJ: Avery, 1985.

Creativity and Healing Websites:

American Music Therapy Association: **www.musictherapy.org**

Dance Movement Therapy: **www.adta.org**

Energy Medicine and Energy Psychology:
www. innersource.net
www.energymed.org
www.emofree.com
www.energypsych.com

Global citizenry: **www.globalcitizens.org**

Healing Story Alliance: **www.healingstory.org**

Humor:
www.humorproject.com
www.aath.org

Meridians: **www.acumedico.com**

Meridian Flexibility: **www. meridianstretching.com**

National Association of Poetry Therapy: **www.poetrytherapy.org**

Storytelling:
Ashley Ramsden: **www.ashleyramsden.com**
Healing Story Alliance: **www.healingstory.org**
Nancy Mellon: **www.healingstory.com**
National Storytelling Network: **www.storynet.org**
School of Storytelling: **www.emerson.org.u**k

Therapeutic Eurythmy:
www.hermeshealth.co.uk
Eurythmy.org

Waldorf Education: **www. whywaldorfworks.org**

Yoga:
www.yoga.about.com
www.abc-of-yoga.com
www.yogabasics.com

Most of the tales in this book are traditional folktales and myths that have been retold and read by generations of storytellers. Recommended, more complete versions of the stories that have been retold in this book can be found in the following:

The Heart
"Who Is More Important" in Eric and Nancy Protter (eds), *Folk and Fairy Tales of Far-Off Lands,* New York: Duell, Sloan and Pearce, 1966.

"Fences or Bridges" in Margaret Read MacDonald, *Peace Tales,* Hamden, CT: Linnet Books, 1992.

"Strawberries" retold by Gail Ross in Jimmy Neil Smith, *America's Favorite Storytellers,* New York: Avon, 1994.

"The Queen Bee" in *The Complete Grimm's Fairy Tales,* New York: Pantheon, 2005.

"The Cottage of Candles" in Howard Schwartz, *Gabriel's Palace: Jewish Mystical Tales,* New York: Oxford University Press, 1993.

The Small Intestine
"Wang-fo, the Painter" in Margaret Yourcenar, *Oriental Tales,* New York: Farrar, Straus Giroux, 1985.

"Healing the Vengeful Sultan" as "King Shahryar and His Brother" in Sir Richard Francis Burton, *The Arabian Nights: Tales from a Thousand and One Nights,* New York: Modern Library, 2001.

The Liver

"The Adventures of Isabel" in Ogden Nash, *Selected Poetry of Ogden Nash,* New York: Black Dog and Leventhal, 1995.

"The Pied Piper of Hamelin" in *The Collected Works of Robert Browning,* New York: Classic, 1900.

"The Myth of Prometheus" in Edith Hamilton, *Mythology,* New York: Grosset & Dunlap, 1963.

"The Elucidation" in Caitlin and John Matthews, *The Encyclopedia of Celtic Wisdom,* Rockport, MA: Element, 2000.

"Jorinda and Joringel" in *The Complete Grimm's Fairy Tales,* New York: Pantheon, 2005.

The Gallbladder

"Two Wolves" in Jack Kornfield and Christina Feldman (eds), *Soul Food: Stories to Nourish the Spirit and the Heart,* San Francisco, CA: HarperSanFrancisco, 1996.

Stephen Vincent Benét, *The Devil and Daniel Webster,* New York: Holt, Rinehart and Winston, 1965.

"The Adventures of Isabel" in Ogden Nash, *Selected Poetry of Ogden Nash,* New York: Black Dog and Leventhal, 1995.

"The Story of the King Hamed bin Bothera and the Fearless Girl" in Kathleen Ragan, *Fearless Girls, Wise Women, and Beloved Sisters,* New York: Norton, 1998.

The Large Intestine

Watty Piper, *The Little Engine That Could,* New York: Grosset & Dunlop, 1976.

Jan Brett, *The Mitten: A Ukrainian Folktale,* New York: Putnam, 1989.

"Living Under Pressure" as "It Could Always Be Worse" in Mary Zemach, *It Could Always Be Worse: A Yiddish Folk Tale,* New York: Farrar, Straus & Giroux, 1976.

Heinrich Zimmer, *The King and the Corpse,* New York: Pantheon, 1948.

"The Image Maker" in Ed Brody, Jay Goldspinner, Katie Green, and Rona Leventhal (eds), *Spinning Tales, Weaving Hope: Stories of Peace, Justice and the Environment,* Philadelphia: New Society, 1992.

The Lungs

"The Girl Who Loved the North Wind" in *Parabola* (Winter 1995).

"The Story Behind the Sorrow" as "Tell It to the Walls" in K. Ramanujan, *Folktales from India,* New York: Pantheon, 1991.

"Br'er Rabbit and Br'er Tiger" in Linda Goss and Marian E. Barnes (eds), *Talk That Talk,* New York: Simon & Schuster, 1989.

"The Legend of Saint Christopher" in Jacobus de Voragine, *The Golden Legend: Readings on the Saints,* trans. William Granger Ryan, Princeton, NJ: Princeton University Press, 1993.

"The Legend of Kuan Yin" in Martin Palmer, Jay Ramsay, and Man-Ho Kwok, *Kuan Yin,* London: Thorsons, 1995.

The Stomach

Paul Galdone, *The Little Red Hen,* New York: Seabury Press, 1973.

Cynthia Jameson, *The Clay Pot Boy,* New York: Coward, McCann & Geoghegan, 1973.

"The Vision of MacConglinne" in Robin Williamson, *Wise and Foolish Tongue*, San Francisco, CA: Chronicle Books, 1991.

Robin Williamson, *The Craneskin Bag,* Edinburgh: Canongate, 1989.

Joseph Jacobs, *More Celtic Fairy Tales,* New York: Dover, 1968.

"Eating the Sky" in Julius Lester, *Black Folktales,* New York: Grove Press, 1992.

"Sweet Porridge" in *The Complete Grimm's Fairy Tales,* New York: Pantheon, 2005.

"Joe and the Button Factory" in *A Virtual Songbook* at www.scoutsongs.com.

The Spleen and the Pancreas

"Coming Down to Earth" told by Pat Bowen.

"Tobias and the Angel" in *The Book of Tobit,* New York: Harper, 1958.

"The Oil of Mercy," the story of Cain, Abel, and Seth, in Jacobus de Voragine, *The Golden Legend: Readings on the Saints,* trans. William Granger Ryan, Princeton, NJ: Princeton University Press, 1993.

The Bladder

"When the Mask Slips" as "Sheronin the Half-Elven," traditional Irish tale, origin unknown.

"Amateratsu" in Pomme Clayton, *Tales of Amazing Maidens,* London: Orchard Books, 1995.

"The Juggler of Notre Dame" in Tomie de Paola, *The Clown of God,* New York: Harcourt Brace Jovanovich, 1978.

The Kidneys

Charles Dickens, "A Christmas Carol."

"King Janaka" in Harish Johari, *The Monkeys and the Mango Tree,* Rochester, VT:
Inner Traditions, 1998.

"The Three Languages" in *The Complete Grimm's Fairy Tales,* New York: Pantheon, 2005.

The Skin
"Love in a Garden" in Blanche L. Serwer-Bernstein, *In the Tradition of Moses and Mohammed,*
Northvale, NJ: J Aronson, 1994.

"Hanner Dyn: An Arthurian Legend," accessed at http://storysocks.pages.web.com.

"The Rattlesnake Story" as "Snake's Jive" in Allison M. Cox and David H. Albert (eds), *The Healing Heart: Communities,* Gabriola Island, BC: New Society, 2003.
"Tales of Finn MacCool" in Rosemary Sutcliff, *The High Deeds of Finn MacCool,* London:
Bodley Head, 1967.

"Allerleirauh" in *The Complete Grimm's Fairy Tales,* New York: Pantheon, 2005.

The Pericardium
"Josel and the Master Builder" as "Warmth of a Fire" in Sharon Creeden, *Fair is Fair,* Little Rock,
AR: August House, 1994; and in Pinhas Sadeh, *Jewish Folktales.* New York: Doubleday, 1989.

"The Faithful Mandarin" as "The Seventh Mandarin" in Jane Yolen, *Tales of Wonder,* New York:
Schocken Books, 1983.

"Ay, Ay, Ay" in Liliane Nérette Louis, *When Night Falls Kric! Krac!: Haitian Folktales,* Englewood,
CO: Libraries Unlimited, 1999.

"The Pear Seed" in Sharon Creeden, *Fair is Fair,* Little Rock, AR: August House, 1994.

The Thymus
"The Bountiful King" retold by Mary Black in David Holt and Bill Mooney (eds), *Ready-to-Tell Tales,* Little Rock, AR: August House, 1995.

"The House of Celebration" in H. Ostermann (ed), *The Alaskan Eskimos* (from the notes of Knut
Rasmussen), Oslo: Norlis, 1941.

"Finn Defends Tara" in Rosemary Sutcliff, *The High Deeds of Finn MacCool,* London:
Bodley Head, 1967.

"The Lotus Eaters," Book IX in Homer's *Odyssey.*

"Paradise Island" in Indries Shah, *World Tales,* New York: Harcourt Brace Jovanovich, 1979.

The Appendix

Ji-Li Jiang, *The Magical Monkey King,* Fremont, CA: Shen's Books, 2004.

"The Cauldron of Ceridwen" in T. W. Rolleston, *Celtic Myths and Legends,* New York: Dover, 1990.

"The Crystal Ball" in *The Complete Grimm's Fairy Tales,* New York: Pantheon, 2005.

The Genitals

"The Creation of the Sexes" in Ruth Finnegan (comp, trans), *Limba Stories and Story-Telling,* Westport, CT: Greenwood Press, 1981.

"The Story of 'No'" in Betty Peck, *Kindergarten Education,* Stroud, UK: Hawthorn, 2005.

"Ye-ma-ha," a sacred oral tradition myth of the Yorisha people.

"Churning the Milky Ocean," in Pomme Clayton (ed), *The Orchard Book of Stories from the Seven Seas,* London: Orchard Books, 1997.

"The Buddah and the Courtesan" in Roy C. Armore and Larry D. Shinn, *Lustful Maidens and Ascetic Kings,* New York: Oxford University Press, 1981.

'The Green Bottle' as "Women" in Milton Rugoff, *Harvest of World Folktales*, NY: Viking, 1968.

"The Graveyard Siren" in Guy de Maupassant, *The Complete Works of Maupassant,* Kila, MT: Kessinger, 1903.

The Brain

Robert Fulghum, *It Was on Fire When I Lay Down on It,* New York: Villard Books, 1989.

"Johnny Whopstraw and the Hare" in Alan Garner, *A Bag of Moonshine,* New York: Delacorte Press, 1986.

"The Donkey" in *The Complete Grimm's Fairy Tales,* New York: Pantheon, 2005.

"Lady Truth" in Jane Yolen (ed), *Favorite Folktales from Around the World,* New York: Pantheon, 1988.

"Theseus and the Minotaur" in Edith Hamilton, *Mythology,* New York: Grosset & Dunlap, 1963.

"Perseus and the Gorgon" in Edith Hamilton, *Mythology,* New York: Grosset & Dunlap, 1963.

"Lucifer's Fall" in Jacob Streit, *And There Was Light,* London: Rudolf Steiner Press, 1976.

Index

fear, 66, 67, 105, 147, 201, 232
fingers, 29, 31, 32, 43, 72, 157, 169, 176, 196, 204, 206
Fisher King, 53, 54
food, 42, 57, 108, 109, 113, 120
forehead, 119, 197, 226
forgiveness, xvii, 178

G
genitals, 209, 220, 221, 250
giants, 28, 091, 227
Gilgamesh, 164
grief, 24, 96, 141, 171
Grimm, Brothers, 25, 43, 110, 151, 185, 204, 228
guilt, 121, 173, 180

H
Hafiz, 19, 71, 085
headaches, 64, 71,
healer, 171, 199, 220
healing, xi, xiii, xiv, 34, 36, 157, 239
heart-protector, 144, 169, 172, 173
hepatitis B, 48
hips, 163, 222
hormones, 117, 185, 197, 210
Hysteria, 34, 40

I
ideals, 21, 75, 76, 241
images, xvi, 36, 92, 153, 170, 232
imagination, xiv, 58, 100, 108, 133
immune system, 36, 135, 161, 164, 184, 185
intelligence, xii, 130, 224
intuitive process, 43

J
Jacob, 125
Jason, 88
Jonah, 199

joy, 28, 159, 188, 202, 217, 218, 230, 234, 240
Jupiter Symphony, Mozart's, 57
justice, 67, 173, 177, 179, 180, 213

K
Kanegis, Bob and Mangual, Liz , 186
kinesiology, xvii
knees, 145, 163

L
Lalla, 32
larynx, 89, 225
leader, 87, 89, 95, 100
leadership, 89, 92,
legs, 72, 73, 169, 196, 209
love, 24, 43, 70, 134, 166, 167, 171, 181
lymph nodes, 117, 184

M
Mars, 65, 173
mask, 130, 135, 138, 140, 141, 248
meditation, 21, 143, 160, 174, 218
Meridian Stretching Center, ix, 119, 172, 196
meridians, xvii
mirror, 99, 136, 155, 221, 224, 233, 233

N
Nasrudin, 136, 202
negativity, 029, 034, 112, 154
Nike, 118
Noah, 145
nose, 104, 196, 225

O
ovations, 132,
Ovid, 136

P—Q
pain, 24, 66, 159, 170, 196, 202
peace, xiv, 21, 25, 83, 122, 123, 152
Pinocchio's nose, 160
Plato, 224
prayer, 52, 97, 169, 181
Prometheus, 52, 053

R
Raphael, 124,
resilience, 28, 43, 117
resistance, 61, 75, 76, 84, 092
Rumi, 28, 147, 202, 211

S
Saint George, 52, 058
Saturn, 117
Scheherazade, 40, 41
School of Storytelling, 133, 246
Scrooge phenomenon, 151
selfless service, 52, 58
Seth, 125
Shakespeare, 67, 97, 125, 146, 211
shaman, 138, 140, 214
Shiva, 81, 83, 84, 216
shoulder, 225
shoulder stand *(Sarvangasana)*, 194, 237
silence, 145, 146, 153, 154, 178
Simpleton, 25, 26, 29
sinus chambers, 89
skull, 223, 226
spine, 118, 129, 130, 144, 145, 169, 225
spiritual nourishment, 119
stars, 132, 154, 155, 211, 229
starvation, 92, 110
Steiner, Rudolf, ix, 200, 229
sun, 24, 52, 136, 155, 166, 217
sweetness, 117, 118, 121, 126, 127